The Complete Guide to Creating Oils, Soaps, Creams, and Herbal Gels for your Mind and Body

101 Natural Body Care Recipes

• • •

Marlene Jones

The Complete Guide to Creating Oils, Soaps, Creams, and Herbal Gels for Your Mind and Body: 101 Natural Body Care Recipes

Library of Congress Cataloging-in-Publication Data

Jones, Marlene.
  The complete guide to creating oils, soaps, creams, and herbal gels for your mind and body : 101 natural body care recipes / by Marlene Jones.
      p. cm.
  Includes bibliographical references and index.
  ISBN-13: 978-1-60138-369-3 (alk. paper)
  ISBN-10: 1-60138-369-X (alk. paper)
  1. Essences and essential oils--Therapeutic use. 2. Beauty, Personal. I. Title.
  RM666.A68J664 2010
  668'.55--dc22
                          2010042082

PEER REVIEWER: Marilee Griffin • EDITOR: Amy Moczynski • AMoczynski@atlantic-pub.com
INTERIOR DESIGN: TL Price • tlpricefreelance@gmail.com
FRONT COVER DESIGN: Meg Buchner • megadesn@mchsi.com
BACK COVER & INSERT DESIGN: Jacqueline Miller • millerjackiej@gmail.com

Printed on Recycled Paper

Printed in the United States

We recently lost our beloved pet "Bear," who was not only our best and dearest friend but also the "Vice President of Sunshine" here at Atlantic Publishing. He did not receive a salary but worked tirelessly 24 hours a day to please his parents.

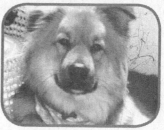

Bear was a rescue dog that turned around and showered myself, my wife, Sherri, his grandparents Jean, Bob, and Nancy, and every person and animal he met (maybe not rabbits) with friendship and love. He made a lot of people smile every day.

We wanted you to know that a portion of the profits of this book will be donated to The Humane Society of the United States. *–Douglas & Sherri Brown*

The human-animal bond is as old as human history. We cherish our animal companions for their unconditional affection and acceptance. We feel a thrill when we glimpse wild creatures in their natural habitat or in our own backyard.

Unfortunately, the human-animal bond has at times been weakened. Humans have exploited some animal species to the point of extinction.

The Humane Society of the United States makes a difference in the lives of animals here at home and worldwide. The HSUS is dedicated to creating a world where our relationship with animals is guided by compassion. We seek a truly humane society in which animals are respected for their intrinsic value, and where the human-animal bond is strong.

Want to help animals? We have plenty of suggestions. Adopt a pet from a local shelter, join The Humane Society and be a part of our work to help companion animals and wildlife. You will be funding our educational, legislative, investigative and outreach projects in the U.S. and across the globe.

Or perhaps you'd like to make a memorial donation in honor of a pet, friend or relative? You can through our Kindred Spirits program. And if you'd like to contribute in a more structured way, our Planned Giving Office has suggestions about estate planning, annuities, and even gifts of stock that avoid capital gains taxes.

Maybe you have land that you would like to preserve as a lasting habitat for wildlife. Our Wildlife Land Trust can help you. Perhaps the land you want to share is a backyard— that's enough. Our Urban Wildlife Sanctuary Program will show you how to create a habitat for your wild neighbors.

So you see, it's easy to help animals. And The HSUS is here to help.

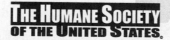

2100 L Street NW • Washington, DC 20037 • 202-452-1100
www.hsus.org

Author acknowledgement:

Special thanks to all my sources who provided me with a wealth of knowledge and made me look good when I could not do it on my own.

Author dedication:

To my sister Jacquie Harakis who, by example, inspires me to continue working toward becoming a healthier person.

To my father, Gordon Dolla, who by his untimely death on Feb. 4, 2010, taught me that when we love, we must articulate.

To my beloved mother, Elizabeth Dolla, for teaching me how the strength and love of a mother can conquer almost all.

To my siblings, Maria Paula, Victor, Debra, and Esther, for allowing me to open my heart to new possibilities.

To my wonderful children, Julian, Jedd, and Jael, for reminding me every day that I am blessed and that mothers must always make time to play and have fun, even while writing a book.

To their father, Steven Jones, for trying to be malleable and allowing me to keep working with him toward success.

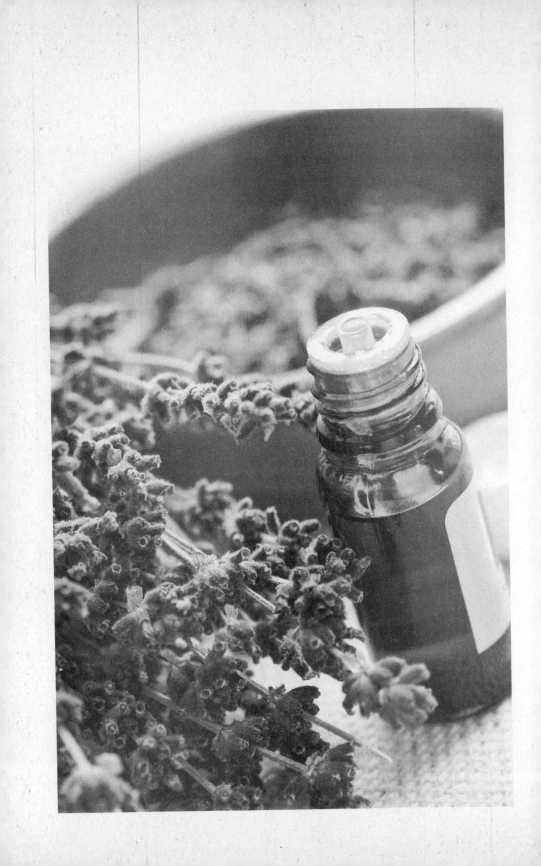

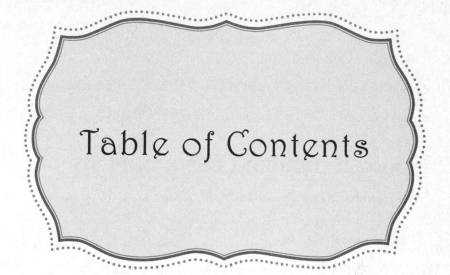

Table of Contents

Chapter 2: Handling Essential Oils   41

Chapter 3: Common Carrier and Base Oils   61

Chapter 4: Common Essential Oils 73

Table of Contents
• • •

Chapter 5: Uncommon Essential Oils 101

Chapter 8: Essential Oils for the Home — 151

Chapter 9: Bath Salts and Oils — 161

• • •

Chapter 10: Making Soap 165

Chapter 11: Methods of Basic Soap Making   199

Table of Contents

• • •

Chapter 12: Beauty and Wellness Treatments 221

Chapter 13: Other Important Uses for Essential Oils   243

• • •

Chapter 14: Quick Guide of Conditions and Essential Oils Used for Treatment   255

Chapter 15: Tools and Further Research   271

Conclusion   277

Glossary   279

Bibliography   281

Author Biography   283

Index   285

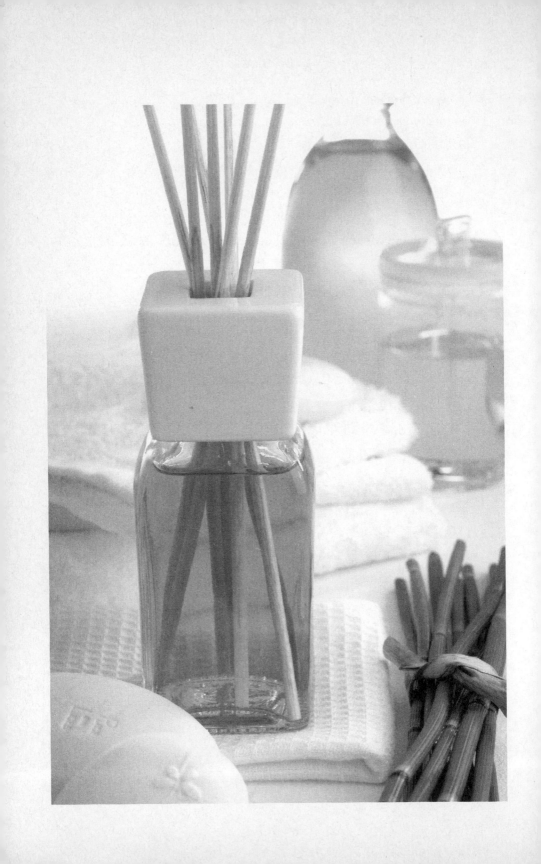

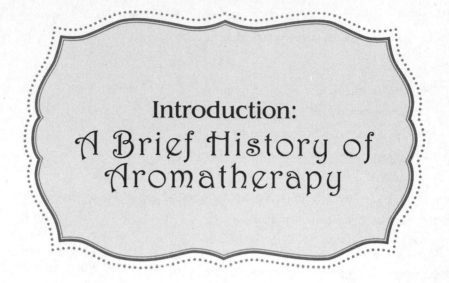

Introduction:
A Brief History of Aromatherapy

If you are like a growing segment of the U.S. population, you care about what you consume, either through ingestion or topically. You care about the fat content in the morning pastry you eat every morning and the synthetic chemicals in the scented body cream you use. You also care about what these products can do to your body — whether they might be responsible for the increasing incidents of cancer across the country, and how you can substitute them for safer products that may enhance and prolong your life.

The increasing popularity of aromatherapy comes from more than just its fragrant qualities. It comes from the enlightenment of those who have, either accidentally or purposefully, gleaned knowledge that nature has healing powers for the body and for the mind. These powers were discovered and used long before the beginning of modern civilization by notorious historical figures like Cleopatra. More than leadership skills punctuated Cleopatra's legendary rule of Egypt. According to David Pybus, a young Cleopatra was able to captivate some of the most powerful men of her time — Julius Caesar and Mark Antony — due to her knowledge and use of natural scents, which were both perfumes and intoxicants. Pybus is a self-described "aromancer," a fragrance specialist, who heads the Scents of Time project. Through this project, he has captured and bottled what he believes are the ancient scents of Cleopatra, Tutankhamun (also known as King Tut), Pompeii, and the Mayans.

"Never underestimate the intoxicating power of the blue lotus," Pybus writes on his website, **www.aquadeluna.com**. The Egyptian lotus (*nymphaea caerulea*) is an ancient flower that was revered by ancient Egyptians, including Cleopatra, who believed it rose and fell with the sun. Part of that reverence might have come from the flower's stimulating effects, which Cleopatra might very well have relied on. Today, the blue lotus is used in aromatherapy and is said to bring about heightened awareness and tranquility.

Cleopatra is the most prominent figure among ancient Egyptians who used aromatherapy. There is no recounting the history of aromatherapy without examining its use in ancient Egypt, as well as in other parts of the world like Africa, Asia, and Europe. Aromatherapy is said to have begun with Cleopatra's Egyptians, who used infusion to extract oils from fragrant plants before using them for medicine, cosmetics, and other uses, including cooking. During infusion, plant matter is soaked for a specific period in oil or another liquid while a gentle heat source, such as the sun, is applied. Infused oil is what remains after the concentrated parts of the plant are loosened during the process and the remaining plant matter is strained from the developing liquid. Infused oil, though not considered pure essential oil, is useful in aromatherapy because it contains concentrated plant essence that can be therapeutic.

Aromatherapy, from the two words "aroma" and "therapy," incorporates the use of olfactory, or smelling, senses. According to the National Association of Holistic Aromatherapy, aromatherapy is "the art and science of utilizing naturally extracted aromatic essences from plants to balance, harmonize, and promote the health of body, mind, and spirit." The oils and scents we derive from plants and flowers help us create and maintain health and happiness, physically, spiritually, and emotionally.

In the Bible, aromatherapy started long before Cleopatra conquered Egypt. According to Kayla Fioravanti, an Aromatherapy Registration Council (ARC) registered aromatherapist, vice president, chief formulator, and co-founder of Essential Wholesale and Essential Labs, there are 188 Biblical references to essential oils. An example of these biblical references is in Exodus 30:22-25: "Then the Lord said to Moses, take the following fine spices: 500 shekels of liquid myrrh, half as much (that is, 250 shekels) of fragrant cinnamon, 250 shekels of fragrant cane, 500 shekels of cassia — all according to the sanctuary shekel — and a hint of olive oil. Make these into a sacred anointing oil, a fragrant blend the work of a perfumer. It will be a sacred anointing oil."

Fioravanti continues to learn about aromatherapy as ARC requires. ARC, now a certified nonprofit based in Oregon, was established in 1999 by the Steering Committee for Education Standards in Aromatherapy. ARC registers and tests qualified aromatherapy professionals with thorough knowledge of the craft.

Hippocrates, who is called the father of modern-day medicine, is widely credited with dismissing the common belief that illness came from supernatural forces. He was born in Greece in 460 B.C. and his life's work is the basis of today's medicine. Hippocrates carefully studied patients' symptoms before prescribing medication and subscribed to the healing power of nature, including the use of herbs. Historical accounts note that during his lifetime, Hippocrates studied and documented more than 200 different herbs; evidence that today's medicine probably began with aromatherapy, which is now considered alternative medicine.

How Smell Works

Imagine you are driving through your suburban neighborhood one morning on your way to work. In the car with you is your 3-year-old who you first have to drop off at day care. As is customary during your weekday morning driving routine, you chat about your surroundings. "Is that a building?" she asks as you pass by a familiar apartment complex. You look forward to the questions she asks you this morning, just as she does on other weekday mornings.

She begins to ask you another question, and you assume that it is another question about the building, but she surprises you. "What is that stinky?"

You look at her through the rearview mirror and chuckle at the small hand covering her nose. You observe that her eyes have begun to tear up and, as if on cue, an offensive smell wafts up your nostrils, causing you to stop chuckling. You recognize the smell of a skunk even before you see the famous foul-smelling critter. It takes more than one minute and a few hundred feet before you stop smelling the contents of the skunk's scent glands.

Though children are not necessarily superb smellers, their sense of smell is more heightened than their other senses. It is highly unlikely that children and even adults think about how their sense of smell works, even though they use it dozens of times in the course of a day. The ability to perceive odors, both pleasant and unpleasant, is often the first reaction people have to stimuli. The ability comes from deep within the nose. Apart from being the gateway to the respiratory system in human beings and other animals, it is a mucus-covered appendage that allows the tiny molecules of a scent to travel to your brain, letting you respond to a smell.

The sense of smell is a chemical reaction that begins when tiny chemical odor molecules float through the air into the nose. Air moves inside the nose, dissolving in the warm, mucus slime that exists within the nose cavern, and allows the chemical molecules you inhale to float upward until they hit the olfactory epithelium — a small ceiling area in the nasal cavity. It contains nerve cells known as olfactory receptor neurons that detect odor.

It is not only odor that dissolves in the thick mucus deep inside the nose. Chemical odor molecules do the same, at least until they reach and get trapped in the limbic system structures, which are considered the most primitive parts of the brain because they influence emotions and memories. Scientists have found that odor molecules perform different functions and nerve cells in the limbic system structures hold on to different smells depending on the shape of the nerve cells. Because odor molecules are trapped within these nerve cells, they are able to tell your brain to sense each different smell you may come in contact with.

Shen notes that each odor molecule affects each nerve independently. For example, he writes "the scent of grapefruit oil, and particularly its primary component limonene, affects autonomic nerves, enhances lipolysis through a histaminergic response, and reduces appetite and body weight." *More information is available at* **www.ncbi.nlm.nih.gov/pubmed/15862904**.

There are involuntary reactions to smell, such as tears streaming from your 3-year-old's eyes after encountering the skunk's scent. Research shows that everyday smells can act as triggers of how your body reacts. For example, the smell of chemicals from paint or smoke has been linked to feelings of fatigue. The smell of rosemary has been linked to boosts in mental clarity and self-esteem, because it stimulates the central nervous system. Chamomile and lavender have been used to stave off hysteria, impatience, stress, and tension.

Current Uses for Essential Oils

Around the home, for aromatic surroundings, first aid, or for a soothing massage, essential oils have a myriad of uses. They can be used to add fragrance to your home by mixing a few drops with water in a spray bottle and using this as an air freshener. They can also be used to clean surfaces in the kitchen or bathroom and used to add fragrance to candles.

Some essential oils are useful for medicinal purposes. For instance, the tea tree oil derived from the leaves of the Australian native narrow-leaved paperbark is a potent antiseptic that can be used for topical treatments for bacterial, fungal, and viral infections, scabies, and even head lice. Next time your child comes home from school with the parasitic insects in his or her hair, try destroying them with some tea tree oil instead of rushing out to your local drugstore.

What You'll Learn

This book will introduce you to the different kinds of essential oils, their characteristics, and their uses. It will show you how they are extracted from their plant bases and readied for use with special equipment that enhances safe handling, which is of utmost importance when handling simple oils, such as lavender, or more complex and toxic oils, like bitter almond.

Considering the amount of work and expense that goes into creating essential oils, learning adequate storage methods that will prolong their shelf lives is very important. This book will show you how to extract, dilute, and protect your essential oils, and how to create and protect soaps, body creams, and herbal gels. You will learn how these natural products can improve your outlook on life. You will also read from experts and professionals who create these products for a living, because they are passionate about the benefits they offer. This learning experience should capture your attention not just because it is interesting, but because it holds the possibility of well-being that can last for the rest of your life. It all starts with essential oils. If you are wondering what they are and how you can use them, please read on.

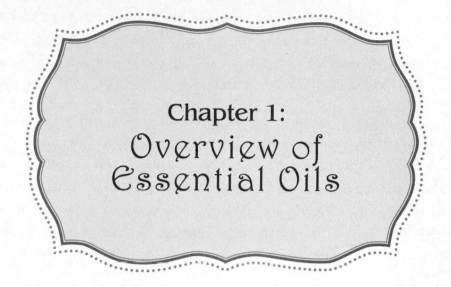

Chapter 1:
Overview of
Essential Oils

What Exactly is an Essential Oil?

Think of a few dozen fresh green leaves from a blooming coriander plant in the palm of your hand. When you squeeze those leaves hard enough, a green, juicy substance will ooze onto your hand. That juicy substance is your basic, undiluted essential oil. The squeeze method of extraction, however, is not one of the methods this book will cover, because it is much more time consuming than any other method featured here. From allspice to lavender and ylang-ylang, everyday and exotic plants are the bearers of essential oils, which, despite their name, do not feel oily. They are called oils because they contain oil-soluble chemicals derived from plant matter.

The term essential oil may vary according to each user, but in this book, the term refers only to the essence — the concentrated and aromatic oils derived from plants and flowers long identified for aromatherapy uses. These oils come from plant leaves, fruits, stems, and roots and are used for a variety of purposes, including therapeutic. You may encounter warnings whenever the therapeutic qualities of essential oils are discussed, advising you not to rely on essential oils to treat serious medical conditions and to seek professional medical care in such cases. It is probably a good idea to follow these well meant pieces of advice while also keeping in mind that essential oils make up the immune systems of some plants, helping them fight infection and repel pests. Imagine then what they can do for you.

Essential oils are classified into three notes or scent characteristics: top, middle, and base. The classification depends on whether their scents are immediately evident once you establish contact with them. Eucalyptus and grapefruit essential oils belong in the top group of oils that tend to evaporate quickly and contain anti-viral properties. They are also light, uplifting, and because they are easily extracted, they are more inexpensive than either middle or base note oils.

A majority of essential oils, like black pepper, cardamom, and rosemary, are classified as middle notes, because they create a balance when blended with other oils. The aromas from middle note essential oils are not always immediately evident but they are characterized by warm, soft fragrances.

Essential oils classified as base notes tend to be heavy with solid aromas like those from balsam of Peru, cedarwood, and cloves. They are intense and rich, making their presence immediately evident when you come into contact with them. They are known to slow down the evaporation of the other oils and are the most expensive of all essential oils.

Because essential oils are **volatile** (meaning that they evaporate quickly) and concentrated, special extraction methods are necessary to separate them from their hosts and harvest them for use. The most common method of extraction is steam distillation, which involves steam cooking the plant to release its essences. Other extraction methods include the following:

- **Expression** — using high pressure to squeeze out plant essences.
- **Enfleurage** — saturating flowers with vegetable oils to release the essences.

- **Carbon dioxide extraction** — using extraction equipment to pressurize and turn carbon dioxide into a liquid that is then used to steam distill essential oils.

- **Solvent extraction** — using chemicals such as alcohol to saturate dainty flowers, allowing them to release their essential oils.

Differences Between Synthetic and Pure Essential Oils

The pure essential oils discussed in this book vary greatly in chemical structure from synthetic essential oils. Pure essential oils come exclusively from plant matter with naturally occurring properties, but synthetic oils contain animal matter, synthetically created oil properties, and naturally occurring oil properties. Using chemical solvents like alcohol is a popular way to create synthetic oil properties. Once chemical solvents have been introduced to plant matter such as leaves or flowers in the extraction process, the occurring oil is called an **absolute** and is not really considered essential oil anymore even though it still possesses some therapeutic qualities. Aromatherapy experts say that even the minutest synthetic component in otherwise pure oil renders it completely synthetic albeit still useful in aromatherapy.

Extraction Methods

Distillation

This is the most common extraction method for essential oils and can include steam distillation, hydrodistillation, or a combination of the two, called water and steam distillation. Water is the common denominator in distillation, but heat plays an important role as well.

In **steam distillation**, an aromatherapist grabs fresh or dried plant matter and a **still** — a contraption similar to a pressure cooker — and starts cooking. Stills range in price from less than $100 to more than $10,000, depending on capacity, whether they can be configured to use electricity, and the materials they are made out of. Stills made out of copper are popular because they reduce sulfur compounds in the final product but are considered to have a negative impact on quality of essential oils. Because of the effects copper has on essential oils, stainless steel stills are recommended. The Essential Oil Company (**www.essentialoil. com**) is a good place to begin shopping for stills and other products used for essential oil extraction.

Hydrodistillation, the oldest method of distillation available, involves tightly packing and fully submerging plant matter in a still's kettle, applying heat of about 212 degrees Fahrenheit, and producing what resembles a pot of soup. A separate still chamber generates pressurized steam that is circulated throughout the plant matter, forcing the plants' cells that contain essential oils to open and release their treasures. As the oils are released, they evaporate and mix with the steam. The still's condenser then cools the steam, allowing it to revert to a liquid state.

Robert Seidel, president of The Essential Oil Company and designer of the "Essencier" essential oil separator, suggests exercising careful calculation once the steam reverts to a liquid state, because there is a continuous flow of watery distillate that has to be separated from the essential oils. This must be done by capturing the water in a separate container while making sure the sill does not overflow and you do not lose any essential oils.

Products like the Essencier can solve the problem because they automatically separate essential oils from the distillates in the still. This allows lighter essential oils to float to the top of the water for easy extraction.

Keep in mind that a few pounds of plant material result in a just a few ounces of essential oils. For instance, more than 8 million jasmine flowers produce just 2 pounds of jasmine essential oil. The good thing is the oils are very concentrated, meaning that a few drops can go a long way.

Expression

Expression is a method of extraction exclusively for obtaining citrus essential oils. Bergamot, lemon, lime, and other citrus fruits are rolled over a trough that has sharp extensions meant to pierce the skin of the fruits and release the oils within. Think of your basic kitchen knife piercing a lemon, releasing the permeating scent of the lemon juice mixed in with essential oils.

Solvent extraction

A rose plant may have thorns, but its flower petals are wispy, sweet smelling, beautiful to behold, and produce some of the most expensive essential oils you can find. Through the use of the solvent extraction method, the essential oils within rose, jasmine, violet, and other delicate flower petals are placed on perforated metal trays before they are sprayed with a solvent that makes them release their essences. Pure alcohol is the solvent of choice because it evaporates, leaving the essential oils behind.

Enfleurage

The enfleurage extraction method, though more expensive than all other extraction methods, is akin to the solvent extraction method. It entails spreading fixed oil, usually vegetable oil or animal fat, onto a sheet of glass mounted on a wooden frame. Flower petals are then placed in the fixed oil before the contraption is placed in the sun and left until the fixed oil is saturated with the essential oils from the flower petals.

A solvent like alcohol is introduced to the petals and once it evaporates, it leaves the essential oils on the sheet of glass. The products of this method are called absolutes rather than essential oils, because using solvents introduces foreign chemical components that render the oil impure in aromatherapy.

Carbon dioxide extraction

Like in the distillation method, carbon dioxide (CO_2) extraction uses high pressure, described in aromatherapy as "hypercritical" at 91 degrees, to extract essential oils. When carbon dioxide is in a hypercritical state, it is neither gas nor liquid. Place plant matter in a stainless steel tank and inject carbon dioxide into the tank. The colorless, odorless gas turns into a liquid, which acts as a solvent on the plant matter. Once the pressure decreases, carbon dioxide reverts back to its gaseous state leaving behind cleaner, fresher essential oils.

Carbon dioxide as a solvent is gaining popularity because no solvent residue remains in the essential oils and the method features no temperature degradation of the oil, which can weaken the essential oils' therapeutic effects.

Precautions When Using Essential Oils

You should make sure to exercise appropriate caution when working with concentrated essential oils. Aromatherapy experts recommend that before attempting essential oil extraction or use, you should have basic knowledge of the oil's qualities, including its scent. Knowing the oil's qualities can help protect children, pregnant or lactating women, and those with underlying illnesses or sensitive skin.

There are a number of "never dos" to observe with essential oils:

- **Never use them undiluted.**

    Using undiluted essential oils can cause permanent skin sensitization, which means becoming allergic to that particular essential oil. In the book *Essential Oils and Aromatics: A Step-by-Step Guide for Use in Massage and Aromatherapy*, Marge Clark, an author and aromatherapy expert who is well quoted in aromatherapy and herbal media stories, shares a personal experience that serves as a great cautionary tale. She shares how she used undiluted lavender oil on broken skin and now suffers from contact dermatitis, a skin sensitivity reaction, if she comes into contact with any form of lavender.

- **Never ingest essential oils except after consulting with a physician or a qualified aromatherapy practitioner.**

Ginger, mandarin, nutmeg, orange, basil, cloves, rosemary, tarragon, oregano, dill, sage, spearmint, cumin, lemongrass … The list of recognizable and safe botanicals essential oils are extracted from can stretch for miles. You can easily find a doctor who can list the benefits of ingesting these botanicals. In fact, you probably have a myriad in your kitchen cabinet.

Still, you should take note that even safe essential oils such as cassia (*cinnamomum cassia*), black mustard (*brassica nigra*), sassafras (*sassafras albidum*), and wormwood (*artemisia absinthium*) can have toxins capable of causing adverse effects if not administered in moderation and with common sense by avoiding ingestion.

- **Never use essential oils on children without a knowledgeable adult present.**

Wanting your child to safely have that famous baby smell is probably something most parents want, and essential oils can help create that. But parents and caregivers should remember that when preparing a blend for a child, essential oils should be doubly diluted. For instance, instead of using 2 drops of essential oil in a mixture, you should only add 1 drop of essential oil in a mixture.

- **Never use them near fire.**

Most common essential oils such as tea tree and lavender have flash points of up to 150 degrees. A **flash point** is the lowest temperature at which a liquid can vaporize into air, forming a mixture capable of igniting.

- **Never use them near the eyes and genitalia.**

  Think of the kind of irritation isopropyl alcohol can cause in a deep cut next time you are considering handling essential oils without protective eyewear or without clothes on. They are especially irritating on mucus membranes and can cause burns in the cornea, which is the transparent part of the eye.

- **Limit sun exposure when using essential oils.**

  Sunlight and high temperatures are known enemies of essential oils, especially those of a citrus nature. They can increase your skin's sensitivity to sunlight, causing you to burn faster and more severely. Experts recommend you should wait at least five hours after using essential oils before exposing your skin to the sun's ultraviolet rays, otherwise you will redden and burn your skin.

- **Label your bottles.**

  Common sense mandates that you should know what is in each dark-colored bottle in your essential oils cabinet both for safety and ease of use. If you have ten bottles of different essential oils in a cupboard somewhere and you are searching for lavender, you do not have to open a number of them before getting to the lavender.

What to Look For When Purchasing Essential Oils

At this point, you know that in order to reap the full benefits of truly natural oils, you should shop for the most natural botanical matter available. A general starting point when purchasing essential oils is to look for pure, undiluted, 100 percent oils.

The following tips should help you have a pleasant shopping experience:

- Keep in mind that because the term "essential oils" is overused in aromatherapy, poor quality oils extracted from poor quality plants and flowers, or oils that are stored poorly and for too long, can still be labeled as essential oils. It is always a good idea to avoid oils stored in clear glass bottles that allow in light, because light is a known enemy to essential oils.

- Essential oil retailers are very common and some are driven only by the need to turn a quick profit — regardless of the effect these oils can have on you and your health. You should be wary of retailers that advertise that they sell to the food and beverage or perfume industries, which require consistent aromas. Consistent aromas can only be created in a laboratory, rendering them non-essential and less therapeutic.

- Do not be overly impressed with words such as perfume oil, fragrance oil, or nature-identical oil because these are most often synthetic oils that are created in a lab and blended with varied but small essential oil amounts. One such retailer, Aloha Bay of Lower Lake, California, has stopped using the label "nature identical" because the company found it to be misleading. The company now prefers to label these oils "nature-identical synthetic scents blended with essential oils" because that is, after all, what they are.

- Seek out vendors who list their products' botanical names. These are those hard to pronounce names, like *eugenia caryophyllata* for clove oil, that tell you the vendor is knowledgeable about aromatherapy. Vendors who list essential oils' origins and method of extraction should also give you a level of comfort that you are purchasing the real deal.

- Avoid vendors who sell each oil for the same price, because it might indicate lax quality and purity. Lavender oil should not cost the same as jasmine or rose oil, which are more difficult to produce and therefore, costlier. Many people tend to be on tight budgets and appreciate "sales," but is it worth saving a few dollars for the valuable health benefits essential oils offer?

- Know there is indication that organic oils are superior to non-organic oils. Organic oils come from plants and flowers grown without pesticides or any other chemicals known to cause adverse health problems.

- Find vendors who test their oils and provide free samples when requested by potential buyers. Some vendors may need to charge a fee for samples, but this shows that they may need to recoup the cost that has already gone into stocking the essential oil.

- Network among potential buyers and with experienced aromatherapy lovers to help find the best retailers. There are aromatherapy mailing lists such as **www.essentialoilslifestyles.com** that can help any budding aromatherapist consumer learn from more experienced aromatherapy consumers.

With these tips in mind, you are well on your way to purchasing pure oils that are as aromatic as they are therapeutic. Before using them, however, you should know how to properly handle them to make sure that you reap the good qualities of essential oils while respecting their potency.

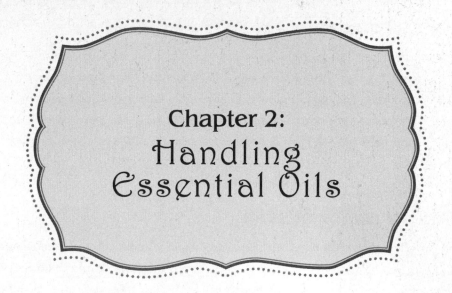

Chapter 2:
Handling Essential Oils

Whether you buy your essential oils from reputable and knowledgeable retailers or you extract your oils yourself from their plant and botanical bases, you will probably realize that each task is time consuming and expensive. You probably would not want the oils contaminated, thereby reducing their shelf lives or impairing their therapeutic qualities. This chapter will walk you through the equipment you need to properly and safely handle essential oils, how and why you need to dilute them, and how to store them.

Equipment for Using Essential Oils

Chapter 1 introduced you to the still, the apparatus used in distillation. But what happens after you have successfully extracted or purchased the high-quality essential oils you desire? You handle them delicately, store them properly, and hope to use them with positive benefits for many days to come.

Therapeutic grade essential oils work best when blended with other oils that can complement and enhance their qualities. For the best quality blends, it is better to not only chose oils that are complementary, but also to have the best equipment that you can afford.

Safety equipment

You already know that you should never handle essential oils without protective gear such as eyewear. To protect your hands during the extraction and even the diluting process, you should also wear disposable latex gloves and perhaps an apron to protect your clothes. Unless you are producing oil on a massive scale and not just for personal use, there is no need for specialized shoes, clothing, or hair covers.

Equipment for blending

Creating an **aromatic synergy**, or blending two and sometimes more essential oils together, can be daunting to a novice, because you must first learn the necessary proportions and which oil combinations create the most powerful blends. Measuring oil drop by drop works well for most people who only blend oil for personal use. Additionally, know that essential oils blend well when they belong to the same note group. For instance, floral oils like jasmine and lavender can blend well to create an uplifting blend that can help calm a stressed mind as you take in this powerful aromatic synergy.

Eyedropper

There is no shortage of retailers and vendors selling eyedroppers for essential oils. The challenge in finding the best eyedropper lies in gauging the correct size. Aromatherapists favor small eyedroppers for most essential oils, because these oils tend to be thin, almost watery in viscosity. Thicker essential oils like sandalwood require larger droppers, but you can also warm the oils slightly by placing them in warm water. Warming these oils will make them thinner and easier to handle.

Measuring Tools

Aromatherapy professionals serving wide client bases might need large scales to measure the right essential oil proportions for blending, but for those people making essential oil blends for personal use, everyday kitchen measurement equipment can work. A teaspoonful of an essential oil of your choice could be the only equipment you need to blend it with another oil and water to make a refreshing house freshener.

Mixing containers

Dark glass containers are always the best to use in aromatherapy, because they are unlikely to include foreign, chemical substances that can alter the fragile composition of many essential oils. These come in varied sizes, from small ones that carry less than an ounce of oil to larger ones that can hold several ounces up to even a gallon of oil. For personal use, smaller bottles will allow you to experiment with different blends for a more potent product.

Storage equipment

Storage containers

You have spent dozens of hours, sometimes in the hot sun and sometimes in bitter cold, tending to your lavender flowers or your eucalyptus plants. Once you have harvested your crop, extracted the essential oils they hide deep within their plant parts, and diluted them with a carrier oil of choice, then you are ready to use them. The question you need to ask yourself here is how long you want to use them — until the bottle is empty or until the oil in the bottle loses all its therapeutic qualities and evaporates?

It is recommended that you store essential oils in dark containers to protect them from harsh light sources that can easily degrade their therapeutic qualities. Aromatherapy experts recommend that you do not buy essential oils with rubber eyedropper tops, because they can cause essential oils to become contaminated because they cause the rubber dropper to dissolve.

Labels

Storing essential oils should open up opportunities for you to be creative and artistic. Herbalist and author Colleen K. Dodt suggests each label, whether handmade or computer-generated, should feature each bottle's ingredients, date of creation, and directions for use in ink that will not smear.

Where to store oils

A general idea is to keep your essential oils out of children's reach, in a high cupboard perhaps, away from bright light, heat, and moisture. The bottles, when not in use, should be tightly closed to keep away contaminants and prolong estimated shelf lives, which can last from three months to two or more years.

Diffusing equipment

Diffusers

Diffusers are considered the most effective and safest way to enjoy the plentiful benefits of essential oils. Diffusers come in many shapes, sizes, and patterns but they work the same way by featuring tubing and a compartment to place a few drops of your favorite essential oils. These diffusers combine air and essential oils to periodically spray fragrant mists throughout the room. They work like air purifiers and most feature timers that allow you to control the level of essential oil concentration in your home or office. Because they work without heat, they will not change the properties of your essential oils. Be prepared to spend at least $50 for a high-quality diffuser.

Alternately, you can use reed diffusers, which feature a bottle inserted with special reeds called rattan reeds that can soak up essential oils in the bottle. Once the reeds are soaked, you can then insert the other end into the essential oil while the already soaked end fills your home or office with aroma. Reed diffusers do not emit soot like candles, so you do not have to worry about having an extra cleaning chore.

Aroma lamps

With starting prices of less than $15, aroma lamps allow you to add your essential oils to any room in your house. Aroma lamps use a candle or electricity to warm the essential oil, which in turn diffuses aroma throughout a room. They should be used with caution and kept out of the reach of children to avoid heat mishaps.

Simmer pots

Just as their name suggests, simmer pots, once they are plugged in, will fill your home or office with the scent of your choice. You can purchase simmer pots from major retailers, both online and in stores, and they can be used with essential oils or dried potpourri, which can be mixed with water and then allowed to simmer for hours.

It is important to exercise basic safety precautions when using one of these items. Citrus essential oils such as lemon are favored for use with simmer pots, because their aromas tend to be uplifting. Do not leave a simmer pot within children's reach or plugged in when you go to sleep or leave the home or office.

Spray bottles

These bottles may come individually or in packages, but spray bottles are a safe and easy way to make sure your clothing and furniture carry your favorite essential oil scent. A general recommendation is that when using essential oils, select dark-colored spray bottles that can also be used to safely store your essential oils, protecting them from the sun's harsh rays.

Dilutions and Solutions

Using a dilution is an effective way to use essential oils without adverse effects. To effectively understand how concentrated essential oils are, imagine a particular essential oil is a brew of tea consisting of 100 tea bags and just enough water to fill a 12-ounce cup. Because one or two tea bags would usually be considered adequate for a 12-ounce cup, the 100 tea bags already brewing would no doubt cause anyone who drinks it to suffer adverse effects that could very well include an upset stomach.

The best way to think of solutions is to once again use your imagination. A large body of water is your **base**, which in aromatherapy are cold-pressed, plant-based oils from vegetables, nuts, or seeds. They are also called carrier oils, base oils, or fixed oils. A smaller body of water represents an essential oil that is more likely to evaporate when temperatures climb up to 100 degrees. Volatility, which refers to the evaporation properties of essential oils, is a common property. However, when they are mixed into the base oil — the large body of water — they are less likely to evaporate and instead combine their properties with base oils to make a more effective and stable body of water.

Difference between dilutions and solutions

Dilution is the process of mixing essential oils with carrier oils that renders essential oils safe to use on skin. Solutions are both the carrier oils used to blend in the essential oils and the final product. Dilutions should differ according to how the finished product will be used and the viscosity, or thickness, of the oil, but it is a safe bet to follow this basic guideline in the dilution process if a healthy, non-pregnant adult will use the finished product: two drops of essential oil to 100 drops of carrier oil, which is known as a 2 percent dilution.

Bear in mind that even with this basic formula, different factors can still make dilution a tricky process. Factors such as the viscosity and temperature of the oil affect how big a drop is. Some oils, such as eucalyptus, are thicker when cold and thinner when warmed up a bit. As such, measuring by the drop is widely acceptable only when creating small topical blends for personal use. Other measuring tools such as a beakers and scales are preferred for larger scale dilutions.

Solutions, sometimes called blended oils, are made up of one or more carrier oils combined with drops of an essential oil. Accurate measurements are necessary to enhance the natural chemical and scent qualities of the solutions.

Aromatherapy experts like Julia Lawless, author of book, *The Illustrated Encyclopedia of Essential Oils*, suggest using a maximum of three essential oils in each solution and experts stress the importance of making solutions with correct concentrations. Some examples of proper dilutions follow:

- A 2 percent solution of two drops of essential oil per 100 drops of carrier oil is great for adult body massage. Conversely, a 1 percent solution of one drop of essential oil per 100 drops of carrier oil would work well for facial massage and should not overpower your olfactory senses or create irritation for your face.

- The notes of essential oils should be factored into any solutions you make. A combination of notes works well, but it is never a good idea to use three top notes together, unless, of course, you are trying to render someone unconscious. They are very intense oils and can give someone a feeling of light-headedness.

Reasons to dilute essential oils

Very few essential oils can be safely used on the skin without dilution. They include lavender and tea tree essential oils. All other essential oils should always be diluted to avoid skin irritation and possibly permanently sensitized skin. For safety, essential oils should be diluted using one or more carrier oils. Essential oils do not lose their therapeutic qualities once diluted, because the structure of the essential oil molecules remains the same.

Common dilutions when using essential oils

Armed with the knowledge of which essential oils blend well with which carrier oils, you should gather your favorite, high-quality essential oil, some dark glass bottles, and eyedroppers so you can make some common essential oil dilutions. Some common cold-pressed carrier oils to dilute your essential oils include: almond, apricot, grapeseed, hazelnut, jojoba, kukui, macadamia, sesame, and wheatgerm.

According to Vanessa Nixon Klein, proprietor of **www.herbsofgrace.com** who has studied and used essential oils for more than a decade, a common dilution pregnant women use is 1 percent, equal to one drop of essential oil to 100 drops of a compatible carrier oil. *You will find other common dilutions as recommended by other experts as you read further.*

Common Solutions of Essential Oils

- Fifteen drops of patchouli essential oil mixed with 1 ounce of olive oil makes great massage oil. For a rich, earthy, masculine scent, make a patchouli tincture — a mixture of patchouli leaves steeped in vodka for several weeks and mixed with water. The amount of water should vary according to each individual's tincture potency preference.

- The right solutions of essential oils make everyday products. Did you know that Vicks VapoRub, Procter & Gamble's topical over-the-counter cough medicine that has been used for decades in many American households, contains eucalyptus oil? You can make your own version of this popular medicine by just adding one drop of eucalyptus essential oil to hot water to relieve your minor colds or achy body.

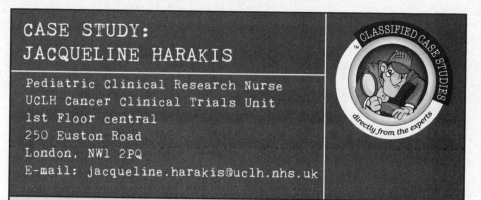

CASE STUDY:
JACQUELINE HARAKIS

Pediatric Clinical Research Nurse
UCLH Cancer Clinical Trials Unit
1st Floor central
250 Euston Road
London, NW1 2PQ
E-mail: jacqueline.harakis@uclh.nhs.uk

"My experience in aromatherapy is very much that of the 'kitchen alchemist' as I create what I use on my skin using ingredients normally found in the kitchen cupboard. Most recipes are accidental, though the Web is a great place to get some tried and tested recipes that can be customized to one's taste and helps take a lot of the messy, wasteful gambling out of the equation.

I find that there are many benefits to aromatherapy not limited to knowing exactly what's going onto my hair and skin and not worrying about 'nasty ingredients' whose long-term adverse effects are unknown. I find that the products I make work as well as, if not better than, commercially made products and they on the whole work out to be cheaper and are genuinely better for us and the environment, too.

There are drawbacks to creating your own products. I find that there is the need to be well organized. I do not use preservatives, so I make small batches, meaning I sometimes run out of stuff and when I am busy I do without for half a day to a day. This drawback is easily overcome though, by making an even smaller batch while I work up to making one that will last a week or two.

My favorite story in creating aromatherapy products happened when I mixed up some aloe vera and oil once and made a lotion. It was a magical discovery. Now, all I do is mix up some aloe vera gel, oil, glycerine, and we have lotion. I add water to dilute if it is too thick and lavender essential oil to add some fragrance.

I recommend simplicity for an average family getting into aromatherapy. When everything is kept simply, any family will discover that virgin oils are fabulous for everything, even for cleansing. Crushed grains and nuts are great for scrubbing the face. Enjoy a piece of fruit and if you can bear it, sacrifice a piece for your face. Wheatgerm or oats and honey are a wonderful facial mask because they are convenient, cheap, and fabulous for the family.

While I do not know how countries compare in their use of aromatherapy, I am aware of a greater number of English and American ladies who are certainly making and using their own cosmetics. Could well be the circles I tend to hang around though, but the United States seems to have greater numbers of people using all natural, organic, homemade products than any other country.

When creating aromatherapy products at home, start small then explore the possibilities. A jar of unrefined coconut oil is amazing for many things — it can be used for a moisturizing bath and as a marvelous body moisturizer. A tube of aloe vera gel, lavender essential oil, and sodium bicarbonate is great for hair instead of shampoo. I even use this to cleanse and scrub my face at least once a week.

Apple cider vinegar and tea tree oil is great for spots. By the way, apple cider vinegar is a must for every kitchen alchemist! Always have a bottle available. Online forums can be a great resource for sharing experiences, but the Skin Deep database website (**www.ewg.org/skindeep**) is wonderful for deciphering the language of cosmetics and checking for the safety of the ingredients in your products there. I love it!"

What Are Carrier and Base Oils?

The safest and most effective way to dilute essential oils is by using carrier oils, which are also known as fixed oils or base oils. They are high-quality vegetable oils derived from nuts and seeds. When mixed with essential oils, carrier oils counterbalance the volatility of essential oils and "carry" essential oils into the skin, thus giving them their name.

Although carrier oils do not have the aromatic qualities of essential oils, they contain vitamins, minerals, and essential fatty acids that make them effective for therapeutic purposes, such as the treatment of conditions like eczema and psoriasis. They are widely used in aromatherapy, making up more than 95 percent of a typical aromatherapy treatment session.

There are several common carrier oils you can use with the most recognizable coming from avocado, almond, apricot, grapeseed, hazelnut, jojoba, olive, macadamia, and sesame. *These oils are discussed in detail in Chapter 3.*

Aromatherapist Sue Charles believes selecting carrier oils is the same as selecting an essential oil because the most important quality is to choose a carrier oil with the most desirable traits for a particular purpose. Sweet almond, for instance, would be ideal for simple body massage other than facial treatments. She said this is because, "some carrier oils contain more of the essential fatty acids and vitamins needed to nourish to the skin and keep wrinkles at bay."

What to consider when choosing carrier and base oils

This is the same as choosing an essential oil. A great starting point is figuring out the properties you need for each particular need you have and researching some basic facts about the oils. Then you can move on to the method of extraction. Any base oil extracted using solvents may not be useful for aromatherapy, because using solvents can alter the oil's nutrient content while introducing foreign qualities. Once this happens, the healing properties of the oils, including antioxidants, essential fatty acids, vitamins, and minerals, might no longer be effective.

Also consider that in aromatherapy, you can allow each aromatherapy blend to speak to your likes, dislikes, and expectations. If you suffer from dry skin, for instance, you would probably choose oil loaded with essential fatty acids like kukui nut oil to help minimize the dryness. If you have dry hair, you may want to choose jojoba oil, because it is similar to sebum from your sebaceous glands, which is your hair's natural oil.

Other points to consider may be fragrance — is it too strong or too light for you? Does it make you dizzy or scatter your mind too much? When considering fragrance, think of the essential oils you are using in the blend and what it adds to the carrier oil.

Processing Methods for Carrier Oils

Carrier oils are just as important in aromatherapy as essential oils. Consequently the quality of carrier oils, just like the quality of essential oils, can determine each blend's therapeutic effectiveness. **Processing** is the act of separating the carrier oils from their hosts. They vary for carrier oils much like extraction methods vary for essential oils, and these methods also determine quality. Cold-pressed carrier oils, for example, are preferred to hot-pressed carrier oils in aromatherapy because their therapeutic properties remain potent and unchanged by heat. Each processing method is discussed in detail below.

Cold pressed

When you want carrier oils to remain in their most natural state, use the cold pressed method of expression. This involves mechanically pressing the fatty portions off nuts and seeds without using heat. To ensure that the end product is in its most natural state, the process mandates temperatures lower than 90 degrees.

Though cold pressing is a difficult method to use to obtain these oils, carrier oils produced using this method are high-quality and suitable for skin care and cooking.

Expeller pressed

This method is similar to cold pressing in that it requires using machinery and force. It differs in that it allows you to use slightly higher temperatures between 120 and 200 degrees with the heat coming from friction generated during the pressing, rather than from an external source.

Because oils that have been expeller pressed may sometimes be expressed using high heat, their natural therapeutic properties may have been compromised.

Solvent extracted

The solvent extracted method of carrier oil extraction involves introducing solvents such as hexane to raw materials. Oil from raw material, like seeds and nuts, dissolves into the solvent, which then evaporates, leaving the oil behind.

The U.S. Environmental Protection Agency (EPA) classifies hexane, a popular solvent in oil extraction, as a Group D product, which is one whose carcinogen effects on humans is unknown. In aromatherapy, however, solvent extraction is unfavorable because solvent traces may be left in the carrier oil, minimizing or destroying its health benefits. Additionally, all nutrients and essential fatty acids usually available in carrier oils are destroyed during the solvent extraction process, rendering them useless for aromatherapy purposes.

Refined and partially refined

Carrier oils derived through refined and partially refined processing have properties that are very different than those you would find in their natural state. The processes, meant to preserve the oils, tend to remove unwanted colors or odors using high heat, freezing, bleaching, and deodorization, all of which damage naturally occurring fatty acids, significantly reducing their therapeutic qualities.

Using partially refined oils is more acceptable in aromatherapy if organic processes are used to derive oils that tend to go rancid faster, like sunflower oil. This is important as long as natural components remain untouched and unmodified during deodorization, winterization, and bleaching.

Unrefined

The unrefined process of extraction uses a screen filtering to remove dust as well as oversized and very small seeds for the finest quality end products, which are generally used in food and cosmetic preparation. The process helps carrier oils retain their rich, dark colors plus strong flavors and scents.

Characteristics of Carrier Oils

Carrier oils have a variety of characteristics that distinguish them from other oils. Unlike essential oils that are always aromatic, carrier oils can be odorless or have nutty aromas. They are also oily to the touch, unlike essential oils, and full of nutrients because they come from within vegetables, fruits, and nuts. As with many vegetables and fruits, carrier oils can quickly go bad if not stored properly. This characteristic is called rancidity and is further discussed below, along with other characteristics of carrier oils.

Nutrients and essential fatty acids

Because carrier oils are from the fatty portions of plants, they are rich in nutrients and fatty acids. Higher levels of saturated fatty acids in oils mean they are more stable, because they do not readily mix with oxygen compared to their counterparts that have higher levels of unsaturated fatty acids.

If you are considering a face lift or think you may be interested in one in the future, consider using carrier oils for bathing, massages, and even cooking. Carrier oils like jojoba contain antioxidants that slow down the oxidative damages in our bodies, thereby keeping wrinkles at bay for longer. Using carrier oils for massage not only makes essential oils easier to work with, but they also act as lubricants, allowing the masseuse's hands to easily and comfortably move on the body.

Carrier oils are very emollient — softening and soothing — making them excellent to use in a bath and massage or on hair. This also applies to those with oily skin who tend to avoid using oil. Oils made from grapes are especially good for oily skin, because they have a drying effect. Vegetable and nut oils are mild and do not require refining. As such, they are usually ready to use even without mixing them with essential oils.

Price

Carrier oils can vary greatly in price based on several factors such as the effectiveness of the raw materials, processing methods, whether organic raw materials are used, and the quantity of oil you are purchasing. More common and versatile essential oils, such as sweet almond oil, are inexpensive, selling for approximately $3 for a 4-ounce container. By contrast, borage oil, derived from the seeds of the borage plant, is more expensive because of its potency. A 4-ounce container can cost $30 or more.

As with all purchasing decisions, you should do your research to make sure you are purchasing from reputable vendors with effective products. It is acceptable to choose not to purchase your oils from any vendor wanting to sell you oils that look like last month's milk, no matter how inexpensive they are.

Organic or non-organic

To decide whether to use organic or non-organic oils, you should first know what organic carrier oils are. Contrary to common misconception, the word organic as referred to in aromatherapy and farming, is not interchangeable with the word natural, and like organic essential oils, carrier oils come from plants that follow strict organic agricultural standards. What exactly is organic, then? The U.S. Department of Agriculture (USDA), which must approve organic labeling as required by the Organic Foods Production Act (OFPA) of 1990, defines organic products as those that emphasize the "use of renewable resources and the conservation of soil and water to enhance environmental quality for future generations." Organic animal products are from animals reared without the use of artificial growth hormones while organic food comes from farms that do not use artificial fertilizers or pesticides.

In aromatherapy, the plants the essential oils come from must pass the USDA standard of organic. There is an ongoing debate about whether organic essential oils have more superior aromas than their non-organic counterparts. The debate first pitted organically grown food and organically reared food animals against those that are grown non-organically.

Barbara Greenwood, a certified aromatherapist based in Canada, said the organic versus non-organic essential oils debate is different from the debate about food because essential oils come from plant matter grown in countries that do not have organic standards similar to those mandated in the United States. "Some plants used for essential oil production are grown and harvested wild where presumably fewer chemicals reach them," she said.

No matter what side of the debate you choose, research has clearly indicated that using synthetic chemicals in food production can result in numerous health issues. For example, a 1996 study by the Environmental Working Group found that 96 percent of water samples taken from 748 towns across the United States contained more than a dozen chemical pesticides, including atrazine. Despite a Cornell University study showing a higher risk of ovarian cancer in female farm workers exposed to atrazine, the EPA determined in 2000 that the pesticide is not likely to cause cancer in humans.

No doubt your decision of whether you should use organic or non-organic essential oils can also come from the fact the organic products cost more. As with essential oils, your decision whether to use organic or non-organic carrier oils should depend on what side of the ongoing organic/non-organic debate you choose.

Color

Carrier oils come in different shades. Some are almost colorless while others are yellow, green, brown, or amber and can sometime mimic the color of the plant material the oil is derived from. Color only matters when the final product you are using the carrier oil for matters to you. For instance, if you are preparing a lavender-based lotion that you want to make a light, almost white color, then you may want to avoid using rose hip carrier oil in the blend, because it is golden red and likely to not lead to a light colored lotion.

Viscosity

Unlike essential oils, carrier oils have little viscosity or thickness. This can be easily controlled depending on how you intend to use them. For example, carrier oils such as olive oil and rapeseed oil are ideal for massage because their viscosity lubricates the skin, allowing them to stay longer on the surface of the skin without quick absorption.

Absorption

Some carrier oils absorb through the skin faster than others and are not the best to use for massage. It is highly unlikely a masseuse wants to keep pouring oil down a patient's back; they would much rather focus on kneading tightly wound tissues to give the patient the relaxed muscles they need. *Chapter 3 has more in depth information on common carrier oils and their absorption levels.*

Shelf life

This ranges from six to 18 months, depending on processing method and available nutrients or fatty acids of each carrier oil. Refined oils and those with naturally occurring tocopherols, like meadowfoam oils, tend to have longer shelf lives. **Tocopherols** are some of the most stable **lipids** (compounds such as oils and waxes that do not dissolve in water) and they are known to be well resistant to oxidization, which can quickly cause oils to become rancid.

Storage

As with essential oils, carrier oils should be stored in dark, tightly sealed containers away from sunlight and indoor lights that can quickly deteriorate the oils. Refrigeration can also help prevent deterioration, which is called rancidity.

Rancidity

Carrier oils may not be as volatile as essential oils, but they are prone to faster oxidization, a process that introduces oxygen to oils, causing them to turn rancid faster, especially when they are not stored properly. Thicker, more saturated and less viscous carrier oils can be stored longer without needing to be refrigerated. You can simply smell your carrier oils to see they have developed rancidity. If it smells different than when you first made it or bought it, do not use the oil.

Aroma

The aroma of carrier oils may not be as pungent as those of essential oils, but they are quite varied, with scents including nutty, herb-like, sweet, warm, and spicy. You will find that each aroma is closely tied to where the oil is extracted. For instance, those extracted from nuts will most likely have a nutty aroma.

Oils to Avoid

Just as you can reap benefits from properly used essential and carrier oils, you can reap unfavorable side effects from certain oils. The following represents a group of the oils you would not want to use for aromatherapy or aesthetic purposes.

Mineral oils

Mineral oil, first referred to in the 1800s as rock oil, is a refined distillate of petroleum. It begins life as crude oil, a yellow-to-black liquid found underground among rocks, and is composed of hydrocarbons. It goes through a complex refining process that uses heat and separation techniques to remove the crude oil's natural color, scent, and taste, allowing it to become either a light liquid or a heavy liquid.

The end products have different properties and are categorized as mineral oil, gasoline, diesel fuel, kerosene, or paraffin. Mineral oil can be further categorized for use in laxatives, baby oil, suntan lotion, ethnic hair products, makeup, lip balms, makeup removers, protective coating for household products, furniture polish, stainless steel cleaners, and for pan and divider oils. In hospitals, mineral-based oils are used to help block the absorption of pathogens that threaten the body's immune system.

Despite the myriad uses available for mineral oils, aromatherapy experts do not recommend them because they do not penetrate the skin and are therefore useless if you are trying to use naturally occurring plant matter to alter mind and body. Some health care providers also recommend that you avoid mineral oil.

Petroleum jelly

Petroleum jelly, most recognizable by the brand name Vaseline, has a number of ingredients such as mineral oils, paraffin, and microcrystalline waxes that come from the "de-oiling" of petroleum. Despite petroleum jelly's popularity, in 2004, the European Union (EU) banned petrolatum, one of petroleum jelly's components, on the premise that it is a carcinogen in breast cancer. Petrolatum is a common impurity of polycyclic aromatic hydrocarbons (PAHs). The impurities come out during the petroleum refining process and have been linked to cancer by several other entities, including the Illinois Department of Public Health, which notes that long-term exposure to PAHs, even in low levels, have resulted in cancer for laboratory animals.

The EU ban notes that petrolatum's "classification as a carcinogen need not apply if the full refining history is known and it can be shown that the substance from which it is produced is not a carcinogen." No such caveat for the industry is available in the United States because petrolatum refined in the country is considered safe. The U.S. Food and Drug Administration (FDA) permits its use in various products such as over-the-counter skin products.

• • •

Instead, if you need a barrier product that works like petroleum jelly, instead of exposing yourself to potential PAHs, use beeswax, a natural wax from honey bees that is available from local beekeepers or online retailers.

Vegetable butters

Vegetable butters come from blending the natural fatty acids of vegetable oils, including stearic acid and monounsaturated oleic acid. Shea butter, which is derived from shea nuts, is a popular vegetable butter. These nuts are cracked and boiled to remove the butter inside, which then undergoes a refining and deodorization process. This process collects unsaponifiable fractions, which are chemical compounds that water cannot break down. These compounds include tocopherols, a common form of vitamin E, that are useful fattening agents in soap making.

Because tocopherols are useful in aromatherapy, you should avoid using vegetable butters that have undergone the process that separates them from their natural hosts. The process can render the part without tocopherols useless for aromatherapy's therapeutic needs.

If your decision is to use none of these products, know that there are many substitute projects you can use. The next chapter covers some of these replacements and the benefits they offer to you.

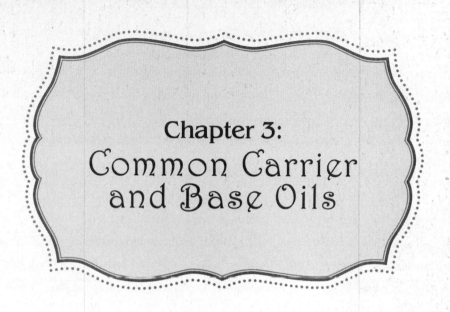

Chapter 3:
Common Carrier and Base Oils

These are oils derived from well-liked, easy to find, and generally inexpensive raw materials. You can use these oils on their own or blend them with an essential oil of your choice. These carrier oils moisturize the skin, while imparting the mind and body therapy that is necessary in aromatherapy.

Apricot Kernel Oil (*Prunus Armeniaca*)

This oil is available from both organically-grown and non-organically-grown apricot kernel, which goes through the expeller or unrefined methods of extraction. It is oily to the touch, has a faint nutty aroma, and can be either light or deep gold in color.

BENEFITS: Aromatherapists recommend it for those with sensitive or prematurely aging skin because of its essential fatty acid contents and vitamins A and E. This oil's shelf life is six to 12 months.

• • •

Avocado Oil (*Persea Americana*)

Avocado oil is available in both organically and non-organically grown avocado, and it is commonly extracted using cold pressing. The refined or unrefined extraction methods can also be used. It is oily to the touch, has a strong herbal odor, and is dark green, especially when unrefined. It has a shelf life of about six months.

BENEFITS: Avocado oil can be used in a variety of products such as bath oils, hair products, and body oils. It has a high content of plant steroids called sterolins that help reduce age spots and heal sun damage and scars. Also high in monounsaturated fatty acids, it has been found to lower low-density lipoprotein (LDL), the bad cholesterol in the bloodstream, while increasing high-density lipoprotein (HDL) the so-called good cholesterol.

The Food Engineering and Biotechnology Department at Israel's Technion Institute of Technology released a study in 1991 acknowledging that avocado oil can increase collagen levels in the skin, which decrease as people get older, allowing the formation of deep wrinkles. And judging by the annual $50 billion-plus cosmetic industry driven by anti-aging products, it is clear to see that many people do not want wrinkles, so many would benefit from using avocado oil during their beauty regiment.

Borage Seed Oil (*Borago Officinalis*)

Derived from the seed of the borage plant using carbon dioxide extraction, this starflower oil, so named for the borage plant's star-shaped leaves, is somewhat oily to the touch. It has light viscosity, has a light to sweet aroma, and a light yellow color.

BENEFITS: A 1993 study from the University of Pennsylvania showed that the fatty acid gamma-linoleic acid (GLA) from borage seed oil is useful in the treatment of rheumatoid arthritis. Other studies have also shown borage oil to be useful on skin conditions such as eczema and flaky skin in infants.

This oil contains alkaloids, which are nitrogen-based natural compounds found in vegetables that can be toxic or sedative. Because of their potential effects on our bodies, borage seed oil is recommended for consumption to the general population in only 1 to 2 gram portions. It is not recommended for pregnant women as it may cause premature labor. It has a shelf life of six months.

Camellia Seed Oil (*Camellia Sinesis* or *Camellia Oleifera*)

This oil comes from the camellia wild flower that is native to Japan and China and the oil is mainly created through cold pressing. It has a sweet, herbal aroma, is pale yellow to golden green with medium viscosity, and has a shelf life of six months to a year.

BENEFITS: Camellia seed oil gains accolades for being the beauty secret of geishas, whose skin no doubt is rejuvenated courtesy of the oil's antioxidants and fatty acids. Another key ingredient, squalene, helps maintain the skin's natural emollient system, minimizing dry skin and premature aging.

Cranberry Seed Oil (*Vaccinium macrocarpon*)

This oil is cold pressed from the cranberry seed. It has a medium viscosity, golden yellow color, and a fruity aroma. Cranberry seed oil has a very stable shelf life and can last for up to two years if stored properly.

BENEFITS: Drink cranberry juice to treat urinary tract infections and use cranberry seed oil as a rich source of omega-3 that lowers bad cholesterol levels

• • •

and promotes healthier hearts. Cranberry seed oil also has oxidative stability, protecting cells from free radical damage.

Evening Primrose Oil
(*Oenothera Biennis L.*)

From the cold pressed seeds of the evening primrose wildflower that grows throughout the United States, this oil is thin with a light nutty aroma and a soft yellow color. Because it is somewhat costly, with a 4-ounce bottle retailing for $13 to $30, it is mostly used in combination with other carrier oils, such as wheat germ for massage, and can even be used for babies with sensitive skin.

BENEFITS: Evening primrose oil has given good results when used to treat a variety of conditions, including rashes, eczema, PMS and treatment of hot flashes, arthritis, diabetic neuropathy, and breast pain, according to the University of Maryland Health Center. The oil is licensed for the treatment of breast pain in the United Kingdom and was found effective at decreasing breast pain in several clinical studies. It has a shelf life of six months.

Fractionated Coconut Oil
(*Cocos Nucifera*)

Considered one of the best multi-purpose carrier oils, it is usually expeller pressed, odorless, viscously light, not oily to the touch, and ranges from a colorless oil to a deep yellow. Because fractionated coconut oil only contains the medium chain triglycerides, a form of fatty acids closer to carbohydrates in structure than fats, it is not considered fully loaded with natural nutrients for aromatherapy.

BENEFITS: Medium chain triglycerides such as fractionated coconut oil function as dietary supplements and are useful for digestive disorders, because they are easily broken down and absorbed into the bloodstream. Fractionated oil is also fully soluble with all essential oils and compatible with soaps. This oil is cost effective and has an indefinite shelf life.

Grapeseed Oil (*Vitis Vinifera*)

Grapeseed oil comes from red, green, and purple wine-making grapes through expeller pressing, partial refining, or solvent extraction. Wine-making grapes can be found in the wild, vineyards, and even in your backyard. Grapeseed oil has a mild taste, mild green color, and almost non-existent scent.

BENEFITS: This oil is great for sensitive skin types and those who do not absorb oil well. Grapeseed oil has also been found in studies to increase antioxidant levels in the blood, aiding in the destruction of free radicals in the body that can cause cell death and accelerate aging.

Hazelnut Oil (*Corylus Avellana*)

Hazelnut oil has a light and nutty aroma. This oil is clear in color and is cold or expeller pressed from roasted hazelnuts. It can have a shelf life of up to a year when stored away from direct sunlight and even longer when refrigerated.

BENEFITS: Hazelnut oil is rich in protein, unsaturated fat, and vitamin B-6 and can be used as a salad dressing. Moreover, the nut is beautiful to behold and because of its high protein content, its oil can help your body regenerate cells, leading to faster wound healing. It also helps tone the skin, leaving users with tight, younger-looking skin.

Hemp Seed Oil (*Cannabis Sativa*)

Cold pressed from the hemp seed, this carrier oil can be golden yellow to dark brown in color with a strong, nutty aroma. This strong color and aroma exists

• • •

because hemp seed oil is unrefined, allowing it to maintain its natural properties. Its shelf life is about one year.

BENEFITS: Hempseed oil has suffered undue unpopularity because of its relation to the illegal cannabis; however, its high levels of proteins and fatty acids make it useful in cosmetics such as lip balms and lotions. It can also be used as an anti-inflammatory massage oil.

Jojoba Oil (*Simmondsia Chinensis*)

This beautiful, waxy liquid comes from jojoba beans through cold pressing. It is mostly odorless but can also have a slight nutty aroma. The oil is golden yellow to brownish liquid with a soft odor and an indefinite shelf life.

BENEFITS: It conditions your hair and scalp and relieves cradle cap, an inflammatory skin condition that causes flaky, yellowish scales to form on an infant's scalp. Cradle cap is said to come from overactive sebaceous glands in the skin that could still be adjusting to the mother's hormones.

Kukui Nut Oil (*Aleurite Moluccans*)

Cold pressed from the kukui nut tree, the official Hawaiian state tree, kukui nut oil emerges as a clear liquid with a light, nutty aroma. With proper storage, you can expect a shelf life of up to a year.

BENEFITS: The oil has been used by native Hawaiians for many decades to protect their skins from salt water, sun, and wind. This oil's ability to quickly penetrate skin makes it excellent for use on dry skin, psoriasis, and eczema.

Macadamia Nut Oil (*Macadamia Integrifolia*)

This cold, expeller pressed, or unrefined carrier oil comes from the macadamia tree and is high in monosaturated fatty acids, palmitoleic acid, and omega-3 and omega-6 fatty acids. It is mostly yellow in color, has thick viscosity, and is oily to the touch. You can expect a shelf life of one year if refrigerated.

BENEFITS: Macadamia is very versatile and is used as an ingredient in cosmetics, snacks, and cooking oil. In aromatherapy, macadamia nut oil is useful in massage, helping heal scars, sunburns, and keeping skin tight and young looking.

Meadowfoam Oil (*Limnanthes Alba*)

A fully bloomed meadowfoam plant is seen as a foamy, solid canopy of creamy white flowers — hence the name. This seed oil, extracted by cold pressing or solvent extraction, has a slight earthy scent, is oily to the touch, and is light golden to medium yellow in color when unrefined.

BENEFITS: Meadowfoam carrier oil contains more than 90 percent fatty acids and tocopherols, which make it resistant to oxidation and good for skin rejuvenation and sunburn protection. As such, it has uses in a number of cosmetic products, including makeup, shaving creams, lotions, body and massage oils, lip balm, as well as hair and nail products. This oil has a shelf life of up to a year with proper storage.

Olive Oil (*Olea Europaea*)

Many well-informed Americans are aware of E-V-O-O, probably because of Rachael Ray, the popular celebrity cook and talk show host. Although it is often associated with culinary pursuits, olive oil, which is thick, green in color, and has a strong olive fruit scent, is useful in numerous other applications such as for skin and hair care. It can be used on its own or in dilution with other carrier oils.

BENEFITS: Olive oil has been documented to control the body's intake of bad cholesterol, which is linked with heart disease. It also activates the secretion of bile and pancreatic hormones, making it useful in ulcer prevention. Olive oil is also useful for soothing rheumatic conditions, and for aesthetic uses in soaps and shampoos.

IMPORTANT NOTE: In 2010, the U.S. Department of Agriculture chose to enforce standards based on science for the use of names such as "virgin" or "extra virgin" in olive oil. This will help consumers differentiate the best olive oil, such as those that are cold pressed, from low-quality impostors that have flooded the market in recent years. This adds to the level of naturalness that aromatherapy calls for.

Peanut Oil (*Arachis Hypogeae*)

Despite consistent reports of allergic reactions to peanuts, the oil derived from this well known nut is important in aromatherapy. Peanut oil has the aroma of roasted peanuts, is thick and clear in color, offers a shelf life of up to a year and contains several beneficial acids, including linoleic.

BENEFITS: This oil is good in general because of its nutrients that include palmitic acid and linoleic acid, which both help increase energy levels. Peanut oil is good for use in massage, because it is emollient and has an oily feel that prevents constant application. It is good for cooking because of its nutrients and is said to be valuable in acne prevention because of its emollient properties. There is debate over whether peanut oil or any other oil can be used in acne prevention, which is said to be exacerbated by oily skin. When in doubt, it is better to consult a qualified aromatherapist or dermatologist.

Pecan Oil (*Carya Pecan*)

This oil is great when added to lavender essential oil and used for massage. It is a light, clear oil with a nutty aroma. The oil contains antioxidants, which are known to decrease the risks of cancer and heart disease as well as delay aging.

BENEFITS: This oil is good to use in massage and leaves the skin moisturized, supple, and young looking. It has a shelf life of 12 months.

Rose Hip Oil (*Rosa Canina*)

Cold pressed or unrefined from the seeds of a rose bush, this oil contains fatty acids like oleic acid that can reduce the levels of bad cholesterol in our bodies, and also contains vitamins A and K. Because it is one of the more expensive oils, it is best mixed with other carrier oils. It has an amber color, watery viscosity, and a slight earthy aroma.

BENEFITS: It increases cell regeneration, allowing it to work especially well on scarred or aging skin to produce new cells. Rose hip also reduces stretch marks, dry skin, brittle nails, and hyperpigmentation, a common problem in those of African origin where patches of skin become darker than the rest of the body after an injury causes excessive deposits of melanin. In Caucasians, liver spots are a common type of hyperpigmentation caused by sun damage.

Sesame Oil (*Sesamum Indicum*)

Sesame seed oil, which is thick in viscosity and is compressed from sesame seed, can sometimes have an overpowering aroma to some users. It is golden yellow to brownish yellow in color and contains vitamins B and E, calcium, and proteins.

BENEFITS: This oil is good to use in massage therapy and is also good to use in cosmetics. Its shelf life is six months to one year.

Sunflower Oil (*Helianthus Annuus*)

This is cold pressed from sunflower seeds. This oil is clear with a tinge of yellow. It has a faint aroma with thin viscosity that does not leave an oily residue. The sunflower carrier oil is loaded with vitamins A, B, D, and E, numerous minerals, and unsaturated fatty acids that break down fat in the body, turning it into useful energy for our bodies while also lowering levels of the bad cholesterol that are known to cause heart disease.

BENEFITS: Sunflower oil absorbs into the skin fairly quickly and is useful in massage. You can expect a shelf life of six months to a year if this oil is stored in cool areas.

Sweet Almond Oil (*Prunus Dulcis*)

This oil is expeller pressed from either organic or non-organic almond kernel. It is very versatile, inexpensive, and a favorite among massage therapists and aromatherapists. It is pale yellow in hue, has a slight almond-like aroma, is of thick viscosity, and contains decent amounts of proteins, fatty acids, glucodides, and minerals.

BENEFITS: This oil works wonders for dry, itchy skin and sunburns. In conjunction with a few other natural ingredients, sweet almond oil makes an incredible body scrub that soothes and calms the skin.

Watermelon Seed Oil (*Citrullus Vulgaris*)

Also known by the more exotic names of ootanga or Kalahari oil, watermelon seed oil is viscously thin, yellow, and has a gentle aroma that is very similar to that of the fruit. The seeds are extracted by hand by pounding watermelon fruits with wooden poles in a wooden bucket. The seeds are then dried naturally in the sun. The oil is more expensive than most carrier oils, is laden with essential fatty acids, and has a stable shelf life of more than two years.

BENEFITS: This oil is very versatile and offers many uses, including as a completely safe alternative to mineral oil-based baby oils, facial oils, hair oils, and massage blends. Additionally, its high linoleic acid content helps your cells hydrate, regenerate, and restructure.

Wheat Germ Oil (*Triticum Vulgare*)

This can be cold pressed or unrefined from the heart of the wheat grain. It is thick with a strong odor and reddish hue. This oil has proteins, minerals, vitamins A, D, and E, and essential fatty acids. It has a shelf life of up to one year.

BENEFITS: This oil blends well with other oils for massage blends and because of its antioxidant properties, it stimulates tissue regeneration, allowing the skin to look younger. It is widely used to get rid of skin dryness and irritation.

Now that you are armed with knowledge of these very useful carrier oils, you are ready to consider their companions. These are essential oils that are commonly divided into two categories — common and uncommon — and they are discussed in the next chapters.

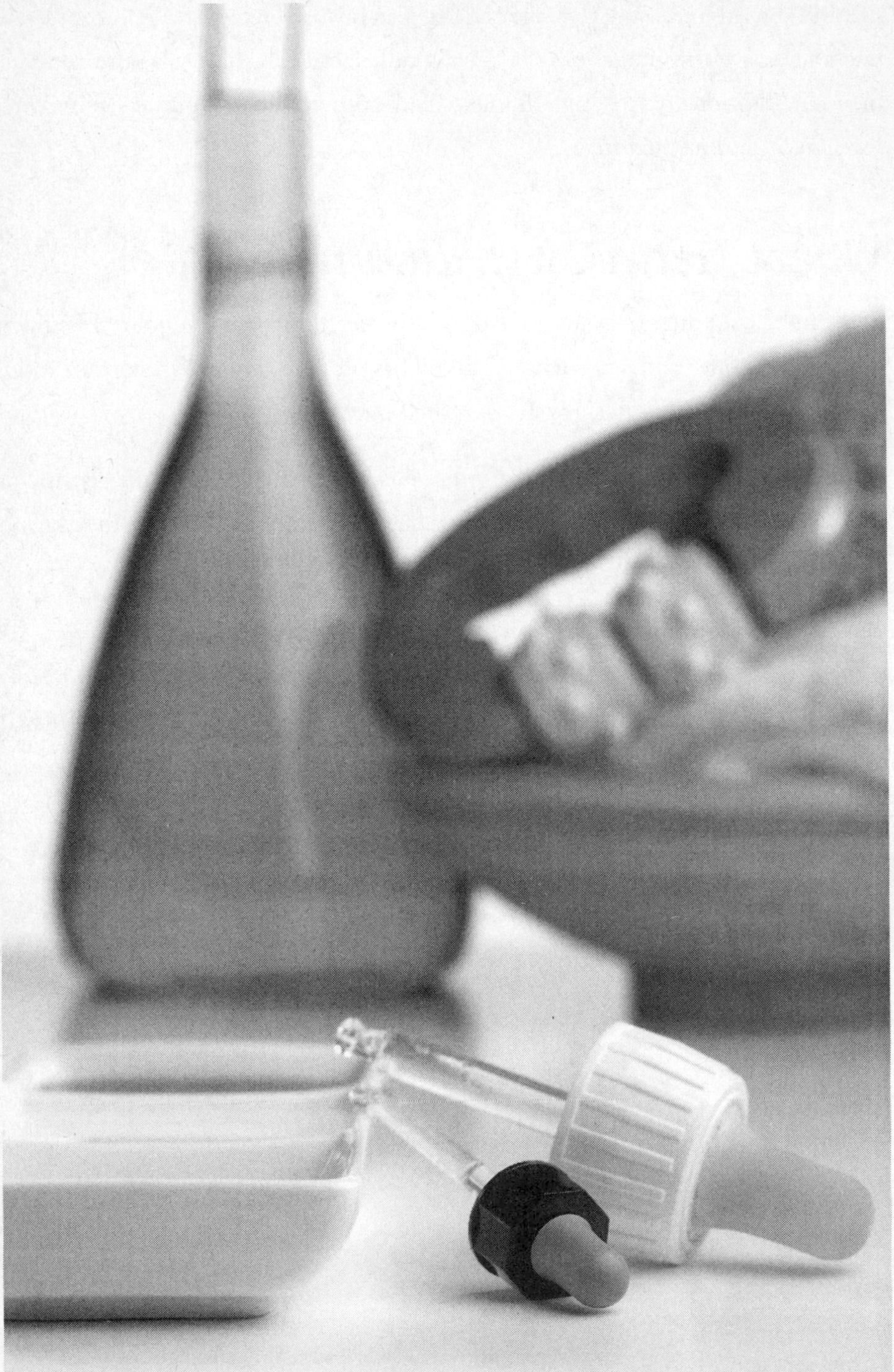

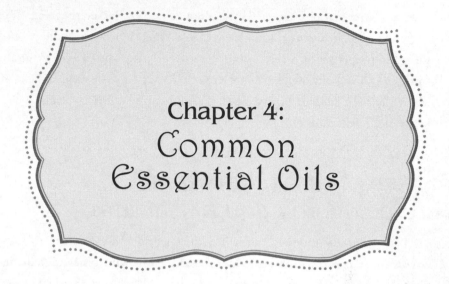

Chapter 4:
Common Essential Oils

The *Journal of Essential Oil Research (JEOR)* (**www.jeoronline.com**) is a respected, scientific resource on the chemical components of essential oils. This journal offers great research on all the essential oils you could ever be curious about and lists the important qualities of these oils, which are extracted from the very essence of plant matter, including plant roots, leaves, bark, and flowers.

This chapter will delve into each essential oil, where it comes from, and its uses. Using well researched information from sources such as JEOR and professional or novice aromatherapy specialists, you will find that each essential oil is different, yet has similar qualities to other essential oils. You will discover the scents, chemical properties, and many uses of both common and uncommon essential oils. At the end of this chapter, you will hopefully be an aromatherapy connoisseur in your own right, ready to delve into the fragrant and therapeutic world of essential oils and aromatherapy in general.

These oils are easy to obtain and tend to be inexpensive with the exception of rose oil and jasmine oil. You will find that many aromatherapy professionals and even essential oil retailers have these oils handy for many uses, as indicated in this chapter.

Note that unlike carrier oils, essential oils do not go rancid. Rather, they evaporate and loose their therapeutic qualities. They have a general shelf life of one to two years if stored properly. The exceptions to this shelf life generality are citrus oils, fir oils, and pine oils, all of which have shorter shelf lives of 12 to 18 months because of a naturally high content of hydrocarbon compounds called terpenes, which result in faster oxidization.

Balsam of Peru (*Myroxylon Pererae, Myroxylon balsamum*)

This is a truly versatile product, but it is a known irritant and allergen to those with sensitive skin when used topically in conjunction with other ingredients. The North American Contact Dermatitis Group (NACDG), an organization that developed to provide support to dermatologists and others while developing information about contact dermatitis (skin inflammation), ranks it as the third most prevalent allergen in the United States. NACDG works in conjunction with the American Contact Dermatitis Society (ACDS), **www.contactderm.org**, which publishes *Dermatitis*, NACDG's home journal.

Balsam of Peru comes from resin found in the bark of the balsam tree that is native to El Salvador but is now common in Central America, including Peru where it was first named. Because of its inviting scent and antiseptic qualities, it has been used in a range of household and beauty products, such as perfumes, deodorant, shampoo, dandruff treatments, household cleaning products, and dental hygiene products.

CHARACTERISTICS

In its natural form, this essential oil is sticky and fragrant. It is classified as a base note and has a woody aroma that has been described as a combination of vanilla and cinnamon. More than 60 percent of its composition is cinnamein and vanillin, naturally occurring chemical compounds in vanilla and cinnamon. Essential oils similar to those in citrus fruit peels also make up part of balsam of Peru's composition.

BENEFITS AND USES

As an essential oil, balsam of Peru is almost unmatched. People have used it topically to ease the discomfort of hemorrhoids, and as an antiseptic for minor wounds and anti-parasitic for ringworms and itch mites. Balsam of Peru has also been successfully used for rheumatism and to relieve coughs and even asthma. Breast-feeding women should not use this oil topically, as it could poison babies.

Benzoin *(Styrax benzoin)*

Like balsam of Peru, this oil is not suitable for those with sensitive skin. The allergy-prone individual may want to avoid topical applications that could result in permanent sensitization to benzoin oil. Benzoin's origins are in the resin of the styraceae tree, which is native to tropical Asia. The resin comes from a "cut" to the bark of the styraceae tree, which after contact with air becomes harder and ready for picking.

CHARACTERISTICS

Benzoin is sweet smelling like vanilla and has been associated with giving a feeling of euphoria, especially when in a citrus mixture. It is classified as a base note and because of its thickness, benzoin is much easier to work with when it is warmed a bit, like in an aroma lamp. When you imagine the fragrance emanating from the lamp, think of the benefits of inhaling benzoin.

BENEFITS AND USES

The benefits of inhaling benzoin when combined with alcohol have been the focus of several studies. The combination, when inhaled, has been found to be especially useful to those suffering from a range of bronchial problems such as coughs, bronchitis, asthma, and laryngitis.

Benzoin also can act as a skin protection against dry lips or bed sores; however, this is a source of debate among aromatherapy specialists. Some do not recommend that benzoin be used in this way because of its concentrated properties and risk of sensitization while others say it is a therapy many people should try. One or several sessions with a qualified aromatherapist who can help you perform a skin test would be useful to determine whether you should use this oil.

Bergamot *(Citrus Bergamia)*

From Bergamo, Italy, this essential oil comes from the fruit rinds of the bergamot tree. The fruit is very much like an orange and releases its essential essences after undergoing the expression process. Like any other essential oil, bergamot oil needs to be stored in an amber-tinted glass bottle. Keep the bottle closed and away from sunlight. If the oil becomes cloudy, this indicates spoilage so do not use this oil.

CHARACTERISTICS

Bergamot essential oil has an invigorating citrus scent. It is classified as a top note and has a light, almost watery viscosity and yellow-greenish hue that mimics the hue of the ripened bergamot fruit.

BENEFITS AND USES

Having digestive or urinary tract issues? Try bergamot. You can also use it to treat psoriasis, acne, or other ailments because of certain elements that come from its components, such as alpha pinene and limonene.

PRECAUTIONS

Limit direct exposure to the sun when using bergamot, because like most citrus fruits, it increases photosensitivity, leaving the wearer susceptible to ugly sunburn and pigmentation.

Black Pepper *(Piper Nigrum)*

Using steam distillation of peppercorns, black pepper oil comes from red, unripened fruit of the piper nigrum plant. The fruits are called peppercorns.

CHARACTERISTICS

It may not make you sneeze, but black pepper essential oil has a sharp, spicy smell that lingers for a while, thus its classification as a medium note. Light in texture, this oil ranges in color from light amber to yellowish green and works well in blends or in a diffuser. You can also use it as an ingredient in massage, bath oils, in a compress, and even in perfume.

BENEFITS AND USES

Black pepper oil has been used as an antiseptic to prevent infection, an antitoxin that can neutralize some toxins, an analgesic for pain relief, an antispasmodic to reduce spasms, an aphrodisiac, a diaphoretic to induce sweating to help reduce fevers, a diuretic to increase urine flow, a laxative, and a tonic to create a feeling of overall wellness. Aromatherapists have also used black pepper oil for muscular aches, fevers, stimulating appetite, and increasing the flow of saliva, which is good for oral health and encourages peristalsis (involuntary muscle contractions that help transport food).

Cardamom *(Ellettaria cardamomum)*

One of the more gentle essential oils, cardamom is steam distilled from the green to brown pellet-like seeds of the leafy cardamom herb that grows well in humid climates and is native to India. The herb itself is useful as a spice and is a fixture in Indian cuisine.

CHARACTERISTICS

This clear to pale yellow oil has watery viscosity and a sweet, spicy aroma with woody undertones. Aromatherapists like it because it blends well with most other oils of citrus and floral nature and with cedarwood, frankincense, patchouli, and sandalwood, among others. Cardamom oil is a middle note.

BENEFITS AND USES

Flatulent much lately? Grab some cardamom. This essential oil is good for digestive ailments and can stimulate appetite, calm the stomach after a vomiting episode, and help with indigestion, heartburn, and diarrhea. Cardamom can also help with general muscular, respiratory muscular spasms, and even teeth whitening.

Cedarwood *(Cedrus Atlantica)*

This essential oil, steam distilled from the wood and sometimes sawdust of the atlas cedarwood tree, can easily be confused with Virginian cedarwood (*Juniperus virginiana*) and Texas cedarwood (*Juniperus ashei*). Cedarwood is best described as an imperial conifer tree, tall — more than 100 feet — and wide. It has been in existence and has been used for thousands of years beginning with ancient Egyptians and Greeks who are said to have used it for embalming and cosmetics. In biblical times, Noah, after surviving the great flood, thanked God by burning cedarwood.

CHARACTERISTICS

The essential oil's aroma is spicy, sweet, and woody. Cedarwood is a base note of medium to thick viscosity, has a yellow to brown hue, and is known to have a drying effect useful in numerous therapeutic applications.

BENEFITS AND USES

Cedarwood, like no other essential oil, uses its astringent properties to help tone up skin by tightening pores, shrinking tissues, and increasing the skin's elasticity. In addition, it acts as an antibacterial antiseptic and is used to treat skin conditions such as eczema and is used in everyday grooming items such as shampoo.

Chamomile *(Anthemis Nobilis, Matricaria Chamomilla)*

This globe-trotting oil is harvested in Rome and Germany and carries the names of both countries: Roman chamomile (*Anthemis Nobilis*) and German chamomile (*Matricaria Chamomilla*). Both are steam distilled or solvent extracted from the flowers of the chamomile plant and have mostly similar medicinal properties, with minute composition differences. German chamomile, for instance, contains the compound chamazulene that works to relieve inflammations and also gives the chamomile its blue color. Roman chamomile, though not as popular as German chamomile, is used as "chamomile lawn" because it can be grown into a thick mat for any garden or lawn. These lawns are common among do-it-yourself projects with directions on how to grow a chamomile lawn.

Remember Cleopatra and the ancient Egyptians? They dedicated this chamomile flower to their sun god and used it in ritual ceremonies to curtail fevers. They were not too far off the mark as chamomile, both in Rome and Germany, has amazing therapeutic effects in a very gentle way as evident in the ever-popular chamomile tea.

CHARACTERISTICS

The flowers resemble daisies and are beautiful when in full bloom. They almost look clustered and have white petals and yellow centers. The essential oil comes out as pale blue oil with a sweet, herbaceous fragrance and light viscosity. Chamomile oil is classified as a middle note oil, because its aroma lingers for more than two hours.

BENEFITS AND USES

Add chamomile oil to your regular massage oil after a difficult workout and instead of grunting in pain, you may just find tranquility for both your mind and body. When your child becomes restless and has trouble sleeping, chamomile can help calm him or her down, giving you both the rest you desperately need. The oil is also used in cosmetics, shampoos, and to alleviate skin conditions like psoriasis, acne, eczema, dry scalp, and rashes. It is also good for the treatment of minor skin inflammations, boils, burns, cuts, and insect bites.

PRECAUTIONS

Those allergic to daisies or those with sensitive skin should refrain from handling fresh chamomile plants to avoid allergic reactions and dermatitis. It is always best to seek the advice of a doctor before using chamomile. In addition, do not use chamomile oil while on anti-coagulant drugs, because it has similar effects and can hinder the drugs' usefulness. Chamomile oil also should not be used by pregnant women, because it has unknown effects on a developing fetus. Those with asthma may develop a sensitivity to this oil and the fragrance can trigger an attack.

Citronella (*Cymbopogon Winterianus*)

Citronella oil maintains its therapeutic properties when steam distilled from the distinctive, tall, tropical grass that grows in Asian countries like Sri Lanka.

CHARACTERISTICS

Its aroma is sharp and familiar — lemony, yet grassy. The citrus nature of its aroma makes it a highly volatile top note, which means that its aroma lingers for no more than two hours. Citronella oil is light in viscosity and blends well with several oils for a variety of uses.

BENEFITS AND USES

Through the use of a diffuser, citronella oil is very useful in keeping away mosquitoes without the use of harsh pesticides during hot, muggy summer nights. The oil can also be used in deodorants, as an antiseptic, a diuretic, and to alleviate colds, headaches, and menstrual irregularity. Citronella acts as an emmenagogue for the latter — a stimulant to make some women regular again.

PRECAUTIONS

Those with sensitive skin should avoid using citronella oil, because it may cause skin irritation. It is also best to avoid it when pregnant to avoid adverse effects on a fetus or if you have underlying health problems that could clash with ongoing treatments.

Clove *(Eugenia caryophyllata)*

Clove oil is steam distilled from the leaves, stem, and flower buds of the small evergreen clove tree with reddish buds that consequently bloom into red flowers. The oil, divided into three subgroups depending on the part of the clove tree from where the oil is derived, is potent and as such, should be used with care to avoid skin irritation.

CHARACTERISTICS

This middle note essential oil is strong with a spicy, woody aroma. It has medium viscosity and is pale yellow color when first distilled. Its color tends to become darker and its viscosity thicker as it ages. Among the clove oil's components is the naturally occurring vanillin, similar to that from the vanilla bean, which adds to its flavor and scent.

BENEFITS AND USES

Clove oil toothpaste may not sound appetizing, but it is a natural mouth freshener and a commonly used dental pain reliever. According to MedlinePlus, a service of the U.S. National Institutes of Health, early studies indicate that clove gel made at home can even be as effective as benzocaine, a topical anesthetic. In addition, clove oil is a widely-used spice and a natural mosquito repellent if undiluted. Therapeutically, it is helpful for indigestion, pregnancy-induced nausea and vomiting, bruises, and burns.

Coriander *(Coriandrum Sativum L.)*

This oil is steam distilled from the seeds of the herbaceous coriander plant, which takes on a spicy aroma after it ripens. The spherical seeds start out green and can turn brown as they age.

CHARACTERISTICS

Coriander oil has a woody, middle note aroma and presents as a thin liquid of clear to pale yellow hue. It contains limonene and can last up to five years with proper storage.

BENEFITS AND USES

Coriander essential oil has plenty of therapeutic qualities. This essential oil can serve as a depurative that removes toxins from the body, an aphrodisiac, analgesic, antispasmodic, deodorant, digestive, fungicide, and stimulant. Coriander oil has been studied for its benefits on mental fatigue, migraines, rheumatism, and muscle spasms.

Clary Sage *(Salvia Sclarea)*

The oil is extracted using steam distillation from the large hairy leaves and the towering purple sage herb plant flowers. The plant is originally from Bulgaria but is now harvested in Morocco, France, and other countries as well.

CHARACTERISTICS

Clary sage is a middle note oil of medium viscosity. It is colorless to pale yellow in color with a floral yet herbal aroma. Like common sage oil, this oil contains thujone, a naturally-occurring substance that is rumored to have "mind-bending" psychedelic qualities but can be toxic if used in excessive amounts.

BENEFITS AND USES

Clary sage essential oil has been used by aromatherapists for a laundry list of everyday problems, including depression and asthma. The oil is also useful as an antidepressant, deodorant, and sedative, as it is known for imparting a sense of euphoria. You can also use clary sage oil for bathing, massages, and soaps.

Eucalyptus *(Eucalyptus Globules, Eucalyptus Radiata, Eucalyptus Citriadora)*

There are several eucalyptus species responsible for different types of eucalyptus oils. They originate from Australia, China, and other countries, and all contain powerful antibacterial and antiviral properties. There are countless species of eucalyptus, but only three are common in aromatherapy, including:

- Sweet eucalyptus (*eucalyptus globulus*) - a perennial with leathery leaves that releases oil used as an antiseptic and stimulant

- Common eucalyptus (*eucalyptus radiata*) - has camphorous (antiseptic) smelling leaves that release the essential oil good for damaged or acne prone skin

- Lemon eucalyptus (*eucalyptus citriadora*) - has lemon smelling leaves that carry the essential oil considered to be calming and antiseptic

CHARACTERISTICS

Eucalyptus essential oils come from the eucalyptus tree and range in color from colorless to pale yellow with a distinct taste and odor that is lemony or medicinal in nature. The thin oil comes from the leaves and twigs of the tree and is classified as a top note.

BENEFITS AND USES

From use in air sprays and vaporization, eucalyptus has given a good measure of protection from infectious illnesses such as influenza. Eucalyptus oil has qualities that prevent or treat sore muscles, inflammation, and spasms while acting as a decongestant, deodorant, antiseptic, and antibacterial. Steam inhalation with eucalyptus has been found to be effective in treatment for colds, easing nasal congestion.

PRECAUTIONS

Beware that fully concentrated eucalyptus oil is poisonous if ingested and pure oil is flammable, so avoid direct exposure. Also, oil contact with the eyes can lead to irritation. Should accidental exposure occur with the eye and other mucous membranes, wash thoroughly with cold water to avoid excessive irritation.

Fir *(Abies Balsamea)*

Think of a Christmas tree when you think of fir essential oil. The oil has been used for centuries and comes from steam distillation of the needle-like leaves unique to the balsam fir tree. Some believe the history of fir essential oil, especially balsam fir, can be traced to biblical days and that the "liquid gold" mentioned in the Bible was in fact balsam fir. Some historians now believe fir oil is the oft-mentioned "Balm of Gilead," a belief reaffirmed when Howard Carter found King Tutankhamun's treasure-filled grave in November 1922.

CHARACTERISTICS

Balsam fir essential oil contains alpha pinene, beta pinene, camphene, and limonene, which makes the essential oil useful for antiseptic capabilities and respiratory infections. It has a citrus-like aroma that smells like lemon and is usually steam distilled from trees saturated with essential oil during cold winter months so the oils can protect the fir needles from freezing.

BENEFITS AND USES

Fir essential oil works well to ease joint pain, muscular pain, rheumatic aches, and inflammation. It has also proved useful in supporting the respiratory system with conditions such as bronchitis, catarrh, chronic coughs, sore throat, colds, and influenza. Balsam fir essential oil is also connected with emotional well-being and stimulating the mind because of its refreshing and uplifting scent.

Ginger *(Zingiber Officinale)*

Ginger is a versatile oil that comes from a root with many uses such as in spices and for tea. Ginger essential oil can bee added to massage and bathing oils. Ginger has pungent, warming, and stimulating properties that, when added to tea or any preferred drink, spreads all over the stomach and then circulates through the rest of the body. Ginger's pungency is attributed to oleoresin, a naturally occurring essence that makes up part of the oil.

CHARACTERISTICS

This essential oil is steam distilled or carbon dioxide extracted from the fresh or dried ground ginger root, sometimes called a tuberous rhizome. The plant is native to Asia and Africa but is now common in all parts of the world. Ginger oil is pale yellow to brown in hue, of medium to thick viscosity, and carries the warm, spicy aroma of the root itself. Ginger oil is classified as a base note, because its aroma can last in a room for many hours and even days.

BENEFITS AND USES

Ginger essential oil works wonders as a digestive aid. Additionally, it has seen many uses in many cultures like the Chinese for diarrhea, rheumatism, and bacterial dysentery. It warms the skin when added to massage oil, making it especially comforting to the body during cold seasons.

Grapefruit *(Citrus Paradisi)*

For a fruit that may have appeared as a horticultural accident that some theorize resulted from crossing a pummelo — a large exotic citrus fruit — and an orange in Jamaica during the 1700s, grapefruit has become quite the hit in aromatherapy. Grapefruit essential oil is cold pressed from the rinds of ripe grapefruits that are first separated from the piths, which are the thick, spongy white layers of the peel. Without extra care, the pith can absorb and decrease the amount of essential oil available for extraction. When this happens, the process has to be repeated in order to extract more oil. This can be time- and money-consuming.

CHARACTERISTICS

One unique factor of this essential oil is its ability to dissolve fat. That feeling you get of slimming down when you eat a citrus fruit is more than a figment of your imagination. Studies have shown that grapefruit essential oil reduces cellulite when massaged into problem areas. It does this by increasing the metabolism of adipose tissue — fat cells in our bodies.

BENEFITS AND USES

Use grapefruit oil for cooking, cleaning, and as a decongestant. It can be beneficial for boosting a sluggish lymphatic system. Grapefruit essential oil, rich in vitamin C, helps in the overall maintenance of healthy skin and tissues and the body's natural ability to absorb iron, which helps guard your body against the threat of infections, from other foods.

Jasmine Absolute (*Jasminum grandiflorum*)

Jasmine essential oil is often extracted from jasmine flowers using the solvent extraction method. Steam distillation is also possible, but, because jasmine flowers are too fragile for steam distillation, solvent extraction is the best method for producing a high yield of oil. Still, because using a solvent to extract the oil introduces foreign substances into the jasmine flowers, there is a risk that the flowers' natural components can undergo a chemical alteration.

Jasmine oil is one of the more expensive essential oils because of the sheer amount of flowers needed to produce it. It is estimated that it takes 1,000 pounds of blossoms — approximately 3.6 million fresh flowers — to produce 1 pound of jasmine essential oil. The flowers have to be collected before sunrise and handled carefully to preserve their delicate scent.

CHARACTERISTICS

Jasmine oil is a very floral, base note oil of medium viscosity. It has a golden tinge to a deep brown color and is very concentrated and potent and should never be used without dilution.

BENEFITS AND USES

Jasmine oil has a wide variety of uses, including stimulating the immune system, destroying bacteria, and balancing dry or oily skin. Beyond that, jasmine essential oil can help with laryngitis, lethargy, immune system stimulation, and helps with feminine issues such as menstrual and labor pains. You can also use jasmine absolute oils in body lotion, shampoo, soaps, antiseptic, and in an oil diffuser as a relaxing air freshener in your home.

Juniper (*Juniperus Communis*)

This oil is steam distilled from the juniper, a tree with stiff needles, small flowers, and berries. The berries produce the coveted essence, but juniper essential oil from only the berries is rare. It is more likely that oil labeled as "juniper berry" comes from the other parts of the juniper tree.

CHARACTERISTICS

With a fresh and woody aroma, juniper essential oil is of light viscosity and colorless to pale yellow hue. Its natural components include pinene, which is a compound that belongs to the terpenes family and can act as a stimulant in the body. These components are credited for giving juniper oil — a middle note — its aroma and structural characteristics.

BENEFITS AND USES

Juniper is popular for treating skin conditions such as acne, dermatitis, eczema, psoriasis, and blocked pores. It is also used for muscle aches and pains, for rheumatism, and as styptic — the powder form of juniper — for stopping minor sore and ulcer bleeds. Juniper oil can help calm down nervousness, treat insomnia, and ease stress.

PRECAUTIONS

Do not use juniper oil during pregnancy, because it can stimulate the uterus and cause premature contractions. Those with severe kidney disease should also refrain from using this oil as it may further irritate the kidneys and cause blood in the urine.

Lavender *(Lavendula officinalis)*

Lavender essential oil is steam distilled from the lavender plant, a woody shrub with beautiful purplish-blue flowers. The name lavender comes from "lavera" the Latin word for "wash," thought to have started because ancient Romans used it in their bath routine.

CHARACTERISTICS

This clear-to-yellow thin oil has a nostalgic, fresh, flowery-yet-fruity scent. It is classified as a top note and has chemical components that read like a chemistry riddle and include limonene and lavandulyl acetate. Its therapeutic properties cannot be doubted.

BENEFITS AND USES

The oil is used as an ingredient in lotions, soaps, body fragrances, bath oils and salts, laundry detergent, and fragrant candles. Because it is steam distilled, lavender essential oil, like other steam distilled essential oils, maintains its therapeutic qualities. Lavender essential oil can be used in treating a long list of problems including acne, itching, flatulence, and sprains.

Lemon *(Citrus Limonum)*

The oil is cold pressed from the peel of lemons harvested from a lemon tree. Its constituents include limonene, responsible for its aroma, and citral, said to aid in digestion, among other things.

CHARACTERISTICS

Lemon oil, like other citrus oils, is classified as a top note. It has a sharp, fresh citrus smell and is pale green or mostly yellow in color. It retains a thin viscosity that belies its potency.

BENEFITS AND USES

The use of lemon goes well beyond a culinary nature. Ever heard of scurvy? It is the vitamin C deficiency now widely known because of popular pirate movies. Because humans lack the ability to create vitamin C, they must rely on fruits and vegetables for this essential nutrient that keeps teeth in place for years to come. Lemon oil used in different applications can help your body maintain the required vitamin C level.

Thankfully, the fruit's high vitamin content that is transferred to the essential oil helps increase the body's immunity against infections. Lemon stimulates white blood cells, which are the body's natural defender against foreign components that seek to inundate it with illnesses. Aromatherapy specialists also note lemon oil's ability to improve circulation in the body. Other health benefits and properties include its ability to alleviate stress disorders, fever, asthma, insomnia, skin disorders, and stomach problems.

Lemongrass *(Cymbopogon citratus)*

This essential oil is steam distilled from the leaves of a fast growing, tall, and fragrant grass that was originally cultivated in India, but now grows in other parts of Asia, Africa, and the West Indies. First popular for its use in several Asian cuisine delights, lemongrass grows well in warm climates but becomes dormant in cold climates. It is more suited for climates such as those found in Florida or California. Lemongrass blends well with a number of essential oils, including lavender, geranium, orange, lime, and bergamot.

CHARACTERISTICS

Although lemongrass is green with hints of yellow, lemongrass essential oil, a top note, is a yellow to brownish thin liquid with a strong, earthy, citrus smell. Lemongrass is an herb very similar to citronella with components that include citronellal, methylneptenone, terpene, and terpene alcohol.

BENEFITS AND USES

With such an array of components, you will find that lemongrass can relieve an equally wide array of problems. In traditional medicine, lemongrass has been useful in combating insomnia, stomach problems, hypertension, fever, skin problems, sore throats, and respiratory problems. It has also been used to eradicate internal parasites.

PRECAUTIONS

Lemongrass essential oil is not recommended for children, for use when pregnant, or if you have a chronic gastrointestinal tract disease, such as stomach ulcers or even esophageal reflux. Aromatherapy experts say that as long it is dispensed in the recommended dosages, it is safe to use. Whenever in doubt, consult a qualified herbalist, aromatherapist, or physician.

Neroli *(Citrus Aurantium)*

This essential oil is also called orange blossom. It is steam distilled from the flowers of the sweet orange tree. Solvent extracted neroli, considered an absolute oil and not an essential oil, is sometimes sold as citrus aurantium.

CHARACTERISTICS

Some aromatherapy professionals classify neroli oil as a top note while others classify it as a middle note. It has a sweet, floral aroma, pale yellow color, and watery viscosity. It includes several chemical components such as a-pinene and b-pinene, both popular alkalis — water-soluble ionic salts – in the fragrance industry.

BENEFITS AND USES

Neroli's effects on emotional well being have been widely documented. It has been documented to lift users out of shock, confusion, nervousness, anger, and mood swings. Neroli oil is also useful in massage and in decreasing the appearances of stretch marks and scars. It can act as an antibacterial, antiparasitic, nerve tonic, and digestive tonic.

PRECAUTIONS

As with most essential oils, neroli, if used neat (undiluted), can result in sensitivity. You should always perform a patch test on a small part of the skin to observe allergic reactions. Pregnant women also should not use this oil unless recommended by a health care provider. Neroli should be used sparingly to maintain a clear head and avoid distractions, as it has sedative qualities.

Orange-Sweet *(Citrus Sinensis)*

Orange essential oil is cold pressed from the fruit's peel. The fruit itself can be categorized into four groups based on geographical ancestry as well as the fruit's unique qualities. The four groups of orange include blood oranges, navel oranges, Mediterranean oranges, and Spanish oranges.

CHARACTERISTICS

Thin and greenish yellow in hue, this oil of watery viscosity and top note classification has the refreshing aroma of fresh orange peels. It has an uplifting quality tied to lifting depression, among other health benefits.

BENEFITS AND USES

Use it in a diffuser to fill your home or office with the sweet orange fragrance or use this essential oil as a relaxing massage oil. Orange essential oil is well known as an anti-depressant that can relax anyone without the mind-altering properties that so many anti-depressant drugs have today. When you become anxious or nervous, orange essential oil can bring you back to a more focused mood. Orange essential oil can treat colds, relieve indigestion and flatulence, reduce phlegm, and can also increase appetite for those suffering from low appetite due to illness. Some aromatherapy specialists also claim the oil can be useful for relieving kidney stones, high cholesterol, and preventing high blood pressure.

For skin care, this essential oil can be used in a massage therapy to help diminish the look of cellulite. It also works wonders on aging skin, which looks younger on those who use it frequently. Other ways you can use this oil include hair products, deodorants, and perfumes. For the home, as evident when you walk down the home care aisle of any grocery store, this oil is versatile in that it can be used in cleaning products. The only difference between these consumer cleaning products and the ones made from natural essential oils are the aromatherapy benefits.

PRECAUTIONS

Follow the general essential oil safety guidelines for this oil and remember to stay out of the sun. If you have questions about how to use this oil, consult with a physician or qualified aromatherapist.

Patchouli (Pogostemon Cablin)

This oil comes from the patchouli tree, a member of the mint family that grows in warm climates. The plant is originally from Asian countries such as Malaysia, India, the Philippines, China, and from South America. Steam distilling the leaves is the most popular method of extraction, but they can also undergo a process that dries and ferments them before they undergo distillation.

CHARACTERISTICS

Patchouli essential oil has a sharp, musky, herbaceous aroma that many herbalists and aromatherapy professionals describe as a hippie-era scent. That description should be laid to rest, because the essential oil's therapeutic qualities stand on their own. The unique patchouli aroma can undergo an aging process that allows it to develop an even deeper, earthier aroma. In fact, aromatherapy specialists note that patchouli essential oil improves the longer it sits. It has an estimated shelf life of three years or longer if stored properly with its color deepening from light yellow to dark brown and its viscosity thickening to a syrup-like consistency or thicker. Its classification as a base note means that its aroma lasts a long time after one comes into contact with it.

BENEFITS AND USES

Folklore has it that English traders in the late 19th century used patchouli to protect Indian cashmere shawls from moths as the shawls made their way to England. Without the patchouli's signature scent, the English would not buy the shawls. Today, patchouli is noted not just for its scent, but also for its numerous therapeutic qualities.

The oil is an excellent topical remedy for skin problems like acne and eczema. It has been used as an antifungal to treat athlete's foot or on hair to get rid of dandruff. Some also credit patchouli with being helpful for healing wounds and diminishing scars. One final use is as a diuretic, allowing a user to urinate frequently and get rid of excess water and salt in the body.

Peppermint *(Mentha Piperita)*

Like patchouli and like its name suggests, peppermint essential oil comes from the mint family. The plant has menthol properties that have been used in candy, chewing gum, cigarettes, breath mints, toothpaste, and mouthwash.

CHARACTERISTICS

Peppermint essential oil, distilled from the freshly cut tops of the mint plant, has a strong, penetrating menthol aroma. The oil also has a sweet undertone to its aroma that is more pronounced when the plant is still young. This oil is a top note that has a clear hue and thin, watery viscosity.

BENEFITS AND USES

Peppermint can be used as an antiseptic, astringent, digestive aid, and decongestant. In massage therapy, it helps stimulate the lymphatic system, a major player in the body's immune system, because it produces immune cells that fight infections. In health treatments, it is also an analgesic that can help relieve sore muscles and joint pain, colic, fever, flatulence, sinus headache, nausea, scabies, and vertigo. In skin care, a very weak dilution can help ease itching.

PRECAUTIONS

Avoid this oil when pregnant or suffering from cardiac fibrillation that results in contractions of cardiac muscles. Peppermint can irritate mucous membranes when taken orally. When used in concentrated amounts, it can constrict the capillaries and cause adverse reactions for those with cardiac fibrillation.

Rose (*Rosa Damascena*)

This can be steam distilled from the petals of the rose flower; however, solvent extraction is also used. Rose essential oil is one of the more expensive products in aromatherapy with ⅛-ounce bottle costing anywhere from $24 to $60, depending on how much rose oil is in a blend.

CHARACTERISTICS

Roses are some of the most recognized flowers around the world. Their gentle aroma is floral and sweet, and it translates well to the essential oil. There are absolute versions of this oil that exist because the flower is too delicate for steam distillation. Some find the absolute has a more "complete" aroma, with more depth true to the rose flower itself. Rose oil is a clear liquid of watery viscosity. It is classified as a middle note and has a medium to watery viscosity. It is a clear liquid.

BENEFITS AND USES

Arabic physician Avicenna is credited with being the first person to distill rose oil. Avicenna wrote a book on the myriad healing properties of rose oil, including as a massage oil, in baths, and in diffusers. It also makes excellent perfume and is gentle enough on the skin to be used without dilution. It can also be used for its stabilizing effects on emotions such as grief, stress, and anxiety.

Rose Geranium (*Pelargonium Odorantissium*)

Rose geranium oil is extracted using steam distillation from the flowers of pink-purple flowers of a bush known to thrive in warm climates like those in its native South Africa. It is not a pure rose in its scent as it has a hint of citrus scent, but it is still used to add the coveted rose smell to fragrances.

CHARACTERISTICS

Light green in color, this thin, middle note oil, when made from the leaves as they start to turn yellow, has a stronger rose aroma than oils made from younger, greener leaves. Suffice it to say that "ripened" rose geranium oil, like ripened fruit, has as stronger smell.

BENEFITS AND USES

Rose geranium oil has been noted to work on the nervous system as a balancing agent that relieves anxiety and stress. Additionally, it removes excess water and salts from the body that can cause high blood pressure and swellings. Other health benefits from the rose geranium oil include curtailing hemorrhaging and treating jaundice and gall stones.

For aesthetic purposes, rose geranium is used in bath oils, lotions, massage oils, and shampoo. Once on the skin, it can help balance sebum secretion while clearing oily skins. It also works well as an antiseptic that is effective in relieving wounds and other skin problems.

Rosemary (*Rosmarinus Officinalis*)

One of the more popular essential oils, rosemary is steam distilled from the leaves of *rosmarinus officinalis*. A few dozens pounds of the leaves create just 1 pound of the essential oil.

CHARACTERISTICS

This oil's clear hue and thin viscosity match its fresh, herb-like, slightly medicinal aroma. Its chemical components include pinene, which can an act as a stimulant in the body. Rosemary can be used for cooking, and in aromatherapy it blends well with other oils that can also be used for cooking, such as bergamot, ginger, orange, lemon, and peppermint. Rosemary oil has a middle note.

BENEFITS AND USES

Rosemary essential oil has many uses, including providing relief to aching muscles; helping joints affected by arthritis or gout; relieving dandruff and other hair care problems; reviving dry, dull skin; and treating exhaustion, varicose veins, muscle cramping, poor circulation, and rheumatism. The oil is also useful in the home as an air freshener.

Rosewood (*Aniba Rosaeodora*)

This oil is steam distilled from the bark and wood of the rosewood, the small evergreen tree also known as *tipuana tipu* that is native to the rain forests of Brazil and other South American countries but is now also used as an ornamental tree in cities around the world. In Brazil, the rosewood tree is considered an endangered species with authorities there requiring that one tree be planted for every mature one that is harvested.

CHARACTERISTICS

The bark of the tree from which rosewood essential oil is extracted is reddish and quite divergent from the oil, which has a slight yellow tinge to it. It is a thin oil with a scent that can be described as mild, warm, spicy, woody, and floral. Rosewood oil is a middle note laden with linalool, a naturally occurring chemical compound now used for several commercial purposes such as to flavor food and to add fragrance to perfumes and household supplies like carpet cleaners.

BENEFITS AND USES

Apart from its uses in the food and fragrance industry, some aromatherapy experts claim that rosewood oil can balance emotions by acting as a natural anti-depressant and an aphrodisiac because its rich floral aroma heightens sexual awareness. Once the oil is diluted with a carrier oil such as safflower oil, it can help alleviate a number of skin issues, including ugly stretch marks, scars, dry skin, acne, and dermatitis. In combination with carrier oil, using 15 drops rosewood to 1 ounce carrier oil, the oil also works great for massage therapy because its volatility is limited.

Sandalwood (*Santalum Album*)

True sandalwood oil is steam distilled from the **heartwood**, part of the root of the increasingly scarce Indian sandalwood tree that is characterized by plenty of green leaves, reddish buds, and flowers. Sandalwood trees are a threatened species in Mysore, India, where the best quality trees are cultivated. These trees have to be under the protection of the country's forestry department officials to protect them from poachers. This makes sandalwood oil expensive.

Another consequence of this tug of war for sandalwood is that the trees are harvested illegally and sold in the black market, making sandalwood oil one of the most adulterated essential oils — more likely to be diluted with synthetically produced oils. Western herbalists now cultivate sandalwood in places like Hawaii in a bid to bypass the instability in India. However, several species grown outside of India differ from the Indian one and are not considered pure sandalwood for aromatherapy purposes.

CHARACTERISTICS

Sandalwood has medium to thick viscosity so when you pour it, it does not flow as freely as water does. It has a rich, sweet, woody scent and a pale yellow hue. Like wine, sandalwood essential oil gets better with age and can maintain its fragrance for years and even decades. Considering that sandalwood trees need to grow for at least 30 years before they are suitable for harvest, you can imagine how rich they can be if left to grow longer.

BENEFITS AND USES

Sandalwood oil, like the tree it is extracted from, has antiseptic properties that make it great for dressing slight wounds. Herbal medicine practitioners in China and the Indian healing science of Ayurveda also use sandalwood oil to reduce anxiety, abdominal pains, chest pains, and relieve genital problems related to sexually transmitted diseases. The beauty and fragrance industry uses it as an ingredient in perfume, shampoo, and soap. In aromatherapy, it works well as a massage oil, in incense, and for skin therapy to ease acne, blackheads, and dry, chapped skin.

PRECAUTIONS

Considering its scarcity, those who care about ethical harvesting should probably find out as much as they can about the sandalwood oil they are considering buying before they actually buy it. Knowledgeable dealers who know where their wares come from can generally give you an idea of where that oil is from and perhaps whether any Indian forestry department officials were injured or killed during the sometimes illegal harvesting of sandalwood. Sandalwood is not considered a spice and should therefore not be ingested or left within children's reach.

Tea Tree (*Melaleuca Alternifolia*)

Tea tree oil got its name from its historical use as a substitute for tea. History has it that while most of the world considered this small tree a weed, Australian Aborigines discovered and began to use it for its healing attributes that are closely connected to its antiseptic properties. Aborigines crushed the leaves and used the resulting paste on wounds. Europe was not introduced to the invaluable oil until the late 1920s, and it was later used in medical kits during World War II.

CHARACTERISTICS

Laboratory studies have proved that tea tree oil has the naturally occurring compound terpinen that has antimicrobial properties useful in the prevention and treatment of infections. The oil is classified as a middle note, is almost water like in consistency, and has a rather pungent spicy-yet-medicinal aroma that belies its pale hue.

BENEFITS AND USES

Studies have found that when applied topically, tea tree oil can reduce the effects of fungal infections such as acne, athlete's foot, and nail and vaginal infections. Tea tree oil has also been found to be invaluable as a topical disinfectant against methicillin-resistant Staphylococcus aureus (MRSA), the strain of bacteria that is highly resistant to any conventional treatment and is commonly found in hospitals, affecting patients with skin lesions, like post-operative wounds and those with depressed immune systems. As with many essential oils, tea tree oil can be added to massage and bath oils. It is also an ingredient in antiseptic creams, lotions, soaps, deodorants, toothpaste, shampoos used for treating scalp conditions such as dandruff and lice, and for pet products used to disinfect fur and skin against parasites.

Vanilla Oleoresin (*Vanilla Planifolia*)

You will find that this oil is mostly solvent — hexane alcohol — extracted from the vanilla bean, which comes from the herbaceous climbing vine that is native to Madagascar. The oil can also be carbon dioxide extracted, which is a more preferred method, because carbon dioxide will not leave any residue that could potentially alter the oil's chemical composition. Solvent extracted vanilla oil is considered an absolute rather than an essential oil.

CHARACTERISTICS

Vanilla oleoresin oil is dark brown and syrup-like in viscosity. It crystallizes when cold but just needs warm water to get it back to its thick consistency. Classified as a base note, the oil has a sweet balsamic, herbal aroma to it and is very different to work with than any other essential oil, because the absolute vanilla oleoresin does not dissolve in carrier oils and will sink to the bottom of any blend. The oil's aroma, attributed to the compounds phenyl esters and vanillin, is the only thing that will dissolve in carrier oils. The inability to dissolve in carrier oils makes vanilla oil recyclable. Each time you use up the carrier oil that rises to the top of a vanilla oil/carrier oil blend, you just add more carrier oil and let it soak up the vanilla oil aroma while the vanilla oil itself remains unused at the bottom of the jar awaiting the next dose of carrier oil.

On the other hand, carbon dioxide extracted vanilla oil will dissolve in carrier oils to make a powerful, aromatic blend. Aromatherapy experts are united in the belief that carbon dioxide extracted vanilla oil has at least ten times the amount of vanillin compared to solvent extracted oil. There is no question that this makes the carbon dioxide extracted oil better for therapeutic aromatherapy purposes than the latter.

BENEFITS AND USES

Vanilla oleoresin can be added to everyday beauty products including lotions, scrubs, bath salts, soaps, and perfumes. The oil is a purported aphrodisiac and calming agent. It also works well in diffusers, aroma lamps, and for massage, even for infants. The use of vanilla is not limited to aromatherapy, however. Its place in the culinary world has been cemented for many years.

Ylang-Ylang (*Cananga Odorata*)

Ylang-ylang essential oil is steam distilled from the long-petaled lemon yellow flowers of the ylang-ylang tree, a tall evergreen tree that is native to Asia. The unusual name for the tree and the oil comes from a Philippine legend about a beautiful young woman named Ilang — flower.

• • •

CHARACTERISTICS

Ylang-ylang essential oil has a very strong, sweet, floral scent that is said to impart feelings of euphoria. To avoid the euphoria, a feeling of intense excitement that may not be suitable in all situations, aromatherapy professionals suggest that you dilute it in carrier oil such as jojoba or almond oil. You can also use it as a blend with other floral oils such as jasmine. The oil, classified as a middle note, is of medium viscosity and is clear with only a slight yellow tinge.

BENEFITS AND USES

Ylang-ylang's euphoria-imparting properties can help calm nervous tension and stress. The oil, made famous by Coco Chanel in Chanel No. 5 perfume, is also favored in other perfumes where it lends its beautiful scent. It is also used in other skin and hair care products.

These common essential oils are complemented by others considered to be less common but still very useful. You will find them in the next chapter and though they are considered uncommon in aromatheraphy, you will probably recognize their names because the plants they come from are more widely recognized for other uses.

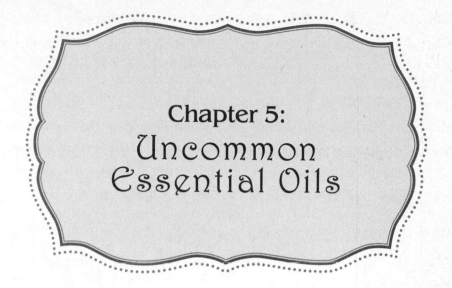

Chapter 5: Uncommon Essential Oils

More than 30 essential oils are listed as uncommon essential oils only because some of the raw materials, like basil, cumin, dill, and lime, are quite popular for other uses and are rarely thought of as aromatherapy tools. Some of them are less frequently used because not much information exists on how to use them safely and effectively.

Allspice (*Pimenta Officinalis*)

Allspice oil is extracted by either water or steam distilled from the berries or leaves of the pimento or pimento tree, a large evergreen tree that is native to the Caribbean islands and especially to Jamaica. The 15th century explorer Christopher Columbus is credited with discovering allspice in the Caribbean islands. He is said to have originally thought it to be the pepper he was looking for and when he took it to Spain, the origin of his journey, it got the name "pimiento," which is Spanish for pepper.

The name "allspice" came about because the tree's aroma is similar to a mixture of at least three spices — cinnamon, clove, and nutmeg. Allspice has been found to have high levels of eugenic, a chemical compound that makes its density greater than that of water. This allows it to saturate the water that develops during extraction and maximize the amount of oil collected.

CHARACTERISTICS

Allspice oil has a sharp, spicy, clove-like aroma. It is classified as a top note essential oil, is viscously thin, and is medium brown in hue. It contains, among other constituents, cineol and methyl eugenic, which contribute to its many uses as an analgesic, anesthetic, antiseptic, carminative, relaxant, stimulant, and tonic.

BENEFITS AND USES

Allspice is popular in men's fragrances. Because of its numerous therapeutic properties, it is used to counter viral and bacterial infections, sinusitis, minor colds, indigestion, and flatulence. A drop of allspice essential oil gently massaged on your chest or any sore area can help relieve congestion, soreness, and stiffness. You can also add allspice to a vaporizer, allowing you to inhale its therapeutic properties that are said to be capable of easing stress.

PRECAUTIONS

The oil's spice qualities make it a likely culprit for irritation of the mucus membranes, especially around the eyes and on sensitive or inflamed skin. Before using allspice essential oil, do a skin patch test to make sure that your skin does not react adversely to its properties. A patch test involves applying a small amount of the oil on your skin and letting it stay for an hour or so while you observe your skin's reaction to the oil.

Angelica Root (Archangelica Officinalis)

This oil comes from the roots of the wonderfully green, herbaceous, and hairy angelica plant that is a perennial native to European countries like France, Belgium, and Holland but is also found in India. The oil is known by several names, including Holy Ghost, archangel, dang gui, and don quai. It is extracted from thick, fleshy roots by steam distillation and is made up of many compounds and consequently has many uses.

CHARACTERISTICS

Pale yellow, sometimes light brown, and of medium viscosity, angelica root essential oil has compounds such as limonene and sabinene that are said to act like calcium channel blockers and work to regulate blood pressure. This essential oil is classified as a middle note and has a strong aroma that is fresh, herbaceous, and peppery at the same time.

BENEFITS AND USES

Angelica root oil has therapeutic, culinary, and cosmetic uses. Chances are that if you like drinking gin or vermouth, you know the taste of the roots and seeds of angelica, which are widely used to flavor such alcoholic drinks. Some cultures, such as the Chinese, considered angelica to have angelic healing powers due to its wide therapeutic uses. You can use this oil as an analgesic, or as a remedy for bronchial ailments, rashes, wounds, rheumatism, headaches, and toothaches.

Anise (*Pimpinella Anisum*)

This is but one variety of anise essential oil. It is extracted from the seeds of the pimpinella fruit, called aniseed. The herb from which the oil is extracted has an umbrella-like appearance and is indigenous to Egypt, Greece, and Turkey. There are two seeds to each fruit of the herb, which has very similar characteristics to the anise star essential oil extracted from the fruit that is discussed later in this chapter.

CHARACTERISTICS

Unlike the plant from which it is extracted, anise essential oil is not dainty. It has been around for centuries and was around during the time of Virgil, the first century author of the epic poem "The Aeneid." Anise is said to have been used in combination with other spices like cumin to make Mustacae, a spiced cake introduced at the end of rich meals as a means to prevent indigestion. In later centuries, similar cakes were brought in at the end of marriage feasts.

The essential oil has a healthy looking yellow hue that makes it look edible — something not suggested — when observed in a clear bottle. It is viscously thin but can crystallize in cold temperatures. Anise is classified as a top note oil and has a strong, spicy, sweet, licorice-like aroma attributed to its naturally occurring compounds that include anethole, camphene, and anisaldehyde.

BENEFITS AND USES

Anise essential oil has many uses that are very different from its use as a culinary flavoring. The oil can be used in making soaps, perfumes, cosmetics, and as an effective bait for mice and other small rodents if smeared on traps. Its therapeutic qualities come from its antiseptic, decongestant, and stimulant properties, making it useful in guarding against and treating skin infections, coughs, and rheumatic conditions.

PRECAUTIONS

Because anise essential oil has narcotic effects if ingested in large quantities, it can slow down circulation and respiration. Care should be taken to ingest it only in professional recommended quantities to avoid these effects. Additionally, the oil is poisonous to small animals and birds and as such, its use with children should be in very limited quantities, or not at all. It can also irritate sensitive skin and cause adverse effects to those with estrogen-based conditions, such as breast cancer, due to the oil's estrogenic properties that mimic the hormone estrogen produced in ovaries.

Anise, Star (Illicium Verum)

This Chinese variety of anise essential oil is extracted by steam distillation mainly from the star-shaped fruits and sometimes from the leaves of the evergreen anise tree that is native to China. Prior to oil extraction, the fruits are harvested before they ripen and later sun dried and crushed.

The herb from which this essential oil is extracted should not be confused with Japanese anise star (*illicium anisatum*), which is quite toxic when ingested and is mainly used to burn as incense.

> **Note:** The Japanese version, which has smaller fruits and a less pungent aroma, is not covered in this book so note that any references to star anise oil henceforth only refers to the Chinese native.

CHARACTERISTICS

Star anise essential oil like anise essential oil has a pale yellow hue, thin viscosity, and the distinctively sharp aroma of licorice. Unlike anise, star anise is classified as a middle note oil. Its aroma is not as strong as that of anise, but the oil blends well with other spicy essential oils like allspice, as well as some with floral oils like lavender and rose.

BENEFITS AND USES

Apart from its uses as a seasoning, as an additive to improve the flavor of medicine and a variety of other compounds including tea, anise star is also credited with alleviating indigestion, flatulence, painful cramps related to menstruation, nausea, colds, insomnia, bad breath, and colic in infants. It is also said to be useful as an expectorant for coughs and for the relief of lice.

PRECAUTIONS

Although the U.S. Food and Drug Administration (FDA) recognizes star anise as a safe herb, pregnant women should avoid using the essential oil, because it can induce spotting, which is bleeding that may signify some sort of fetal distress, and miscarriages usually begin with spotting.

• • •

In 2003, the FDA issued a warning cautioning consumers against the consumption of teas containing star anise after reports noted contamination with the toxic Japanese star anise and consequently myriad side effects in those who consumed the teas. These side effects included hypothermia, convulsions, seizures, spasms, vomiting, and overall feelings of being ill. Although it is still not clear if these effects were from the Chinese star anise or the Japanese star anise, patients with disorders such as epilepsy should probably avoid using Chinese star anise as a general precaution.

Basil (*Ocimum Basilicum*)

Whether you grow your own herbs in your kitchen, somewhere on your property, or you mostly just scoop them up from supermarket veggie shelves, chances are that you are familiar with basil and the prominent role it plays in cuisine, especially Italian cuisine. But did you know that there are two primary types of basil? There is the one you will find at the supermarket and in aromatherapy houses, *ocimum basilisum*, also known as sweet basil, and its close relative, *ocimum sanctum*, also known as holy basil. The latter, just as its name suggests, is used in religious ceremonies in countries such as India and China.

The basil plant is leafy with budding flowers and is typically no more than 3 feet tall. It originated in the tropics of Asia and Africa but is now cultivated around the world. Basil essential oil is steam distilled from the plentiful green leaves and sometimes from the flowers.

CHARACTERISTICS

Basil, which contains several compounds like limonene and citronellon, produces an essential oil that is very watery and has a pale yellow to greenish color. The oil is classified as a top note and has a fresh, light, and peppery aroma.

BENEFITS AND USES

Cooking benefits aside, the aroma of basil oil is so refreshing that it gives the allure — some say reality — of clearing the mind of most everyday stressors, restoring mental alertness, and even sharpening one's sense of smell. Additionally, the oil can be used in massage to relieve sore muscles; in burners and vaporizers to benefit respiratory problems, such as bronchitis and sinusitis; digestively to alleviate constipation and nausea; and to help regulate and relieve menstrual irregularities and cramps.

PRECAUTIONS

If you are pregnant or younger than 16, avoid this oil because it can cause stupor and cause these groups of people to fall or have accidents while operating heavy machinery like cars. Additionally, avoid basil oil if you have sensitive skin as it may cause irritation. A simple patch test is a good way to determine your reaction to its spice properties and other constituents, which include estragole.

Note of caution: Estragole, a natural basil constituent, and the subject of laboratory studies, has been found to be associated with cancer in small animals. Human study has not found a similar occurrence.

Bay (*Pimenta Racemosa*)

Bay essential oil, sometimes called sweet bay, Mediterranean bay, or West Indian bay, is steam distilled from the leaves from the *laurus nobilis* or bay laurel tree, originally cultivated in the West Indies and Guyana but now also cultivated in Algeria, Turkey, Spain, and Morocco. The tree has square-like stems, leaves that are opposite each other, and flowers that form whorls or spirals around a single node.

CHARACTERISTICS

Chavicol and methyl chavicol, both bay constituents, are credited with giving the essential oil its herb-like yet fruity aroma. The middle note oil with a deep golden yellow hue has medium viscosity, making it slightly thicker than water.

BENEFITS AND USES

Bay leaves, where the bay essential oil comes from, are a staple spice in French and Creole cooking. Add in just one bay leaf to a pot of spicy shrimp Creole and you may not be able to put your fork down. The oil is also useful for colds, sprains, rheumatism, dandruff elimination, perfumery, and soap making.

Cananga (*Cananga Odorata*)

This oil is steam distilled from the long-petaled, mostly yellow flowers of the cananga tree, a tall tropical tree than can grow 60 feet or more. Cananga is another name for ylang-ylang that is a native of Asia. Top Tropical aromatherapy expert Tatiana Anderson writes on the company's website (**www.toptropicals.com**) that the distillation process, which can last up to 14 hours, is what differentiates cananga from ylang-ylang. Approximately 200 pounds of flowers sealed in a copper jar with 15 gallons of water produces "about 1 to 2 liters (or 1 to 2 quarts) of oil with the most intense aroma" called ylang-ylang extra, according to Anderson. When the process is repeated with the same raw materials, a lower-grade oil called "ylang-ylang oil" is produced. A third distillation process produces cananga essential oil. The various gradations of concentrated aroma are numbered one, two, and three. The distillation produces oil called "cananga oil" used in fragrant soap manufacturing.

CHARACTERISTICS

The oil is of very thin viscosity, ranges in hue from pale to dark yellow, and has a strong, exotic floral aroma that makes it a top note. It tends to blend well with other floral essential oils like jasmine and rose.

USES AND BENEFITS

The name ylang-ylang, said to mean "flower of flowers" in the Philippine language of Tagalog, is associated with young love and as such, cananga essential oil is often used as an aphrodisiac in Malaysia. The story is that cananga fresh flowers were strewn on the beds of newly married couples to help them have an unforgettable wedding night. Cananga oil is used in soap making and is said to have antiseptic and sedative properties that can be useful in treating small cuts or relaxing a tired brain.

Carrot Seed (*Daucus Carota*)

Carrot seed is steam distilled from the seeds of wild carrot, often considered a weed and sometimes called "Queen Anne's Lace" because the flower head, with several white flowers, has a lace-like appearance. It is named for its origins in England and its popularity during the reign of Queen Anne. Some, including the Carrot Museum in the United Kingdom, conclude that the plant is a member of the carrot family, while other herbalists have concluded that it is a member of the parsley family.

CHARACTERISTICS

Worried this oil will have you smelling like carrots and attracting rabbits each time you step out of your home? Do not worry, because it hardly smells like carrots. Its many constituents like cadinene and linalool are responsible for giving it its woody aroma, middle note properties, pale yellow hue, and watery viscosity.

BENEFITS AND USES

Carrot seed essential oil is one of the few oils that can be used on the skin without first being diluted. It can be blended with other essential oils to make perfume and is also safe for daily ingestion to cleanse the liver. Carrot seed oil can also liven dry, dull, and mature skin or remove the yellowish and sickly color on the skin caused by jaundice, a condition that causes the liver to fail in its role to break down the copious amounts of bilirubin it secretes.

• • •

Catmint (*Nepeta Cataria*)

Any plant named Plant of the Year by the Ohio-based Perennial Plant Association (PPA), a professional trade association of herbalists that provides "education to enhance the production, promotion, and utilization of perennial plants," must have some exceptional qualities. Specifically, according to PPA, these plants have to satisfy a number of criteria such as being suitable for a wide range of climate conditions, being of low maintenance and not requiring constant nurturing, pest and disease resistance, easy propagation, and serve a "multiple season of ornamental interest." Catmint, whose leaves, stems, and flowers produce catmint essential oil via steam distillation, was awarded this honor in 2007 when PPA members nominated and voted for its benefits over at least three other nominated perennial plants. The leaves, seeds, and stems of the catmint plant are covered with **trichomes**, which are microscopic bulbs that store the essential oil until they burst after maturity.

Because catmint essential oil is commercially attractive for its insect repellent properties, solvent extraction and enfleurage extraction is sometimes also used. There have been inventions of extraction equipment submitted for U.S. patents, including Patent 20100034906 on the steam distillation of catmint essential oil by a trio of inventors who claim their invention increases oil yield by 13 percent more than traditional distillation equipment.

CHARACTERISTICS

Catmint essential oil contains dihydronepetalactone, a naturally occurring constituent that exhibits insect repellent properties and is responsible for giving catmint its mint-like, herbacious aroma. Sometimes called catnip, catmint oil has sedative effects and is famous for inducing euphoria in domesticated cats. The oil is classified as a middle note and has a very pale yellow, almost clear, hue and medium viscosity.

BENEFITS AND USES

Mosquitoes and cockroaches have been found to respond poorly to catmint oil, which is a plus for most people worldwide who cannot tolerate the painful, itchy bites of pesky mosquitoes or the inevitable filth of cockroaches. The American Chemical Society (ACS), a professional association of chemists, has accepted papers indicating that dihydronepetalactone is more powerful than diethyl-meta-toluamide (DEET), a popular insect repellent found in everyday over-the-counter sprays. Catmint leaves have also been used in tea, and the oil is useful for the treatment of colds, fevers, flatulence, menstrual cramps, migraines, and the reduction of hairball formation in cats.

PRECAUTIONS

Although the FDA classifies catmint as a drug of "undefined safety," there have been no adverse side effects related to using the oil in reasonable quantities. In high ingestion doses, it can cause upset stomach. Households with pet cats should note that when felines inhale too much of the oil, or consume parts of the plant, they are likely to roll on the ground and drool. This is not a harmful or deadly state. It can even be comical, although some cats may not like the feeling.

Cinnamon Bark (*Cinnamomum Zeylanicum*)

This essential oil is steam distilled from the dried inner bark of shoots that grow from the base of the cinnamon tree, a tropical evergreen tree indigenous to Africa and to Asian countries like Burma, Comoro Islands, India, Indochina, Madagascar, and Sri Lanka. The tree that can grow up to 50 feet tall is characterized by a thick bark, strong branches, oval leaves, and diminutive yellow flowers.

CHARACTERISTICS

Cinnamon bark essential oil contains methylhydroxychalcone (MHCP), a compound credited with helping reduce blood sugar levels in diabetes patients. It is a top note with a sweet, warm, spicy aroma that may evoke nostalgic feelings of the holiday season when the use of cinnamon spice is frequent.

BENEFITS AND USES

Though useful for many aromatherapy purposes, cinnamon bark oil is rarely used on the skin because it is a strong irritant. If used externally, the oil blends well with other essential oils like cedarwood, citrus oils, and frankincense for use near mucous membranes, like around the eyes, which are more prone to irritation. Its therapeutic purposes remain intact when taken orally to benefit the digestive, circulatory, rheumatic, and immune systems. It is better used in diffusers to add aroma to your home or office. The aroma is said to reduce headaches and other pains, relax tight muscles, and relieve drowsiness, irritability, and menstrual cramps.

Cumin (*Cuminum Cyminum*)

Cumin essential oil is steam distilled from the seeds of the cumin fruit or pod that comes from the cumin plant. The plant is a native of the Mediterranean, specifically Turkey and India, but now is a common house herb used for cooking. The cumin plant has an umbrella-like appearance with small white flowers. The seeds are harvested when brown and ideally dried before the oil is extracted.

CHARACTERISTICS

Cumin oil, like cumin spice, has a slightly spicy, musky scent attributed to cuminaldehyde, one of its natural constituents. It is classified as a base note because its aroma lingers in the air for hours before it is readily absorbed into the bloodstream and later secreted through sweat. This phenomenon is easily detected in people of Mediterranean or Indian descent who consume cumin as a spice with curry in many traditional dishes. Cumin oil is of medium viscosity and has a deep yellow, almost brown, hue.

BENEFITS AND USES

Used in a 50 percent dilution of high quality olive oil, cumin essential oil can make a very good massage oil capable of imparting its strong therapeutic properties that include being a diuretic, antiseptic, detoxifier, and a stimulant. It is good for the digestive system by acting as a carminative, efficiently pushing sometimes painful gases away from the intestines and preventing further formation of gases. The oil promotes bile discharge from the liver through the small intestines. It also promotes the secretion of gastric juices in the stomach and stimulates contraction of the intestines that allows regular bowel movement.

Additionally, the aroma of cumin can act as an appetizer for those who may be ill or just picky eaters, and it may also nudge the nervous system to help with lethargy. One former use of cumin and cumin oil was as currency to pay taxes by the biblically-famous pharisees.

PRECAUTIONS

Moderation is important when using cumin oil, because too much of it and its smell can cause headaches and nausea in some. The oil also shows properties of photo toxicity when exposed to sunlight, so you should refrain from exposing your skin to sunlight for lengthy periods after an external application of cumin. These recommendations can be universally applied but are more so stressed for pregnant women who may have underlying health needs not compatible with cumin properties.

Cypress (*Cupressus Sempervirens*)

Cypress always is very reminiscent of the Middle Eastern country of Lebanon maybe because of the biblical references of Lebanon and cypress such as in Isaiah 14:8: "Even the cypress trees rejoice over you, and the cedars of Lebanon, saying, 'Since you were laid low, no tree cutter comes up against us.'" The cypress tree is world famous and is native to many parts of the world, including Africa, Europe, the Mediterranean, and the Middle East. It is flame-shaped, grows tall — upwards

• • •

of 70 feet — and has dark green needle-like leaves from which cypress essential oil is steam distilled.

The tree is very hardy. In fact, the second part of the oil's botanical name, "sempervirens," is a Greek word that means "lives forever." As far as legends go, the cross on which Jesus Christ was crucified was partially made out of cypress.

CHARACTERISTICS

Cypress oil has a fresh, herbaceous, pine-like aroma that is very refreshing. The oil has many constituents like cadinene and linalool that are responsible for giving it its middle note aroma, its pale yellow hue, and watery viscosity.

BENEFITS AND USES

The term vapor therapy deftly applies when cypress essential oil does wonders for the chest and nose of anyone suffering from congestion. Use it in a diffuser and inhale its unparalleled refreshing scent to tackle colds and other slight respiratory ailments. About five drops of the oil in your bath water in combination with a carrier oil like jojoba, or about 15 drops in each ounce of your massage oil, can also serve the same purpose. Used this way, the oil has the additional role of acting as a detoxifier, removing excess waste from the lymphatic system and decreasing excessive perspiration.

This incredibly versatile oil also acts as a toning agent for the skin, reducing cellulite and large pores for smooth skin. You can find the oil in soap making, in lotions, colognes, air fresheners, hair treatments, and laundry products.

Dill (Anethum Graveolens)

Dill is widely used as a spice to enhance dishes, but it also holds dill essential oil, which is extracted from either crushed dill seeds, fruits, or the whole herb plant by steam distillation. The herb is a native of Asia but has origins in ancient Egypt and Rome where it was called "anethon" and used as a charm against witchcraft.

You can recognize growing dill by its green feathery leaves and umbelliferous (umbrella-shaped) small yellow flowers and diminutive if compressed seeds.

CHARACTERISTICS

Dill is a middle note oil that smells like grass; has a thin, watery viscosity; and a pale yellow hue. Its main component is carvone, found more plentifully in the oil obtained from the fruit and is somewhat identical to caraway oil, but it is also a beneficial essential oil.

BENEFITS AND USES

Dill oil can be blended in lotion or cream for a therapeutic blend that can help heal wounds. It is also used to promote proper digestion and reduce flatulence and constipation. Use it for vapor therapy to relax and calm the mind or to alleviate coughs and colds.

Fennel (*Foeniculum Vulgare*)

Fennel essential oil is extracted by steam distillation from the crushed seeds of the fennel herb, a native of Egypt characterized by an umbrella-like shape and small, yellow flowers. The oil obtained from crushed seeds is sometimes referred to as "sweet" fennel oil to distinguish it from "bitter" fennel oil that is obtained from a combination of the crushed seeds and/or the whole herb. Sweet fennel oil is the preferred oil for aromatherapy because of its high levels of phenylpropanoids — compounds produced by plants in response to hostile environmental conditions like drought, pollution, infections, and wounding.

CHARACTERISTICS

Apart from phenylpropanoids, fennel essential oil is laden with other natural components like limonene, trans-anethole, and methyl chavicol that contribute to its strong, spicy aroma, sweet licorice-like taste, clear hue, and thin viscosity. Limonene contributes to the oil's aroma, and trans-anethole contributes to its sweetness; it is said to be more than ten times sweeter than sugar. Methyl chavicol contributes to its hue and strong aroma as well, making fennel oil a well-used ingredient in perfumery. Fennel is classified as a top- to middle-note oil.

USES AND BENEFITS

Fennel seeds have been used in the culinary world for centuries, but they, and the essential oil within them, have a variety of other uses in aromatherapy, cosmetics, and folk medicine. The health benefits of fennel oil are partly attributed to phenylpropanoids and they contribute to the oil's antiseptic, anti spasmodic, carminative (for relief of flatulence), diuretic, expectorant, laxative, and stimulant properties.

The trans-anethole properties of fennel oil make it attractive in several industries for flavoring spices, alcoholic drinks, mouthwash, and confectionaries like whipped chocolate. The limonene is said to increase the levels of liver enzymes that can help detoxify the body of carcinogens, which are cancer-causing compounds. Methyl chavicol contributes immensely to the oil's therapeutic qualities. Use the oil at least weekly and you will probably keep cellulite and wrinkles at bay.

PRECAUTIONS

The component trans-anethole is known to boost levels of estrogen, which, though useful for lactating women, can be harmful in pregnant women who already have high levels of estrogen. This can also be harmful in those suffering from cancer of the breast and the uterus and who may already be suffering the effects of high estrogen levels, which is sometimes linked to the cause of such cancers.

Additionally, high levels of methyl chavicol have been found to be a possible carcinogen in small animals even though its use in humans is considered safe. In heavy doses, fennel essential oil may cause narcotic-like effects, resulting in convulsions and hallucinations so those with a history of epilepsy should avoid it.

Frankincense (*Boswellia Thurifera*)

Frankincense oil, like myrrh its biblically-famous counterpart, is a resin — dried sap — obtained from trees that are native to Somalia. Frankincense comes from the deciduous *boswellia thurifera*, which belongs to the Burseraceae family and sheds its leaves annually. When in bloom, the tree is considerably leafy with oblong leaves that alternate toward the tops of the tree's branches. Placing a deep incision on a part of the tree's trunk that has been stripped of its bark allows a milk-like sap to ooze out.

This is just the beginning of a long process that can take three months from start to end, because the sap oozes slowly and is allowed to harden on the tree by exposing it to air before the original incision is later deepened. In three months, the sap usually has attained the required degree of consistency, hardening into yellowish tear-shaped oleo gum resin that is scraped and carried away in baskets. After this, the oil is extracted by steam distillation.

CHARACTERISTICS

Frankincense essential oil is a base note with a woody, balsamic-yet-spicy smell. It has a pale yellow to pale green hue. Also, bear in mind that because frankincense oil comes from tree sap that tends to be very thick, it is very viscous. The oil's components include incensole acetate, which is said to lower anxiety.

BENEFITS AND USES

Although frankincense oil is widely used in aromatherapy for its aroma in incense burners, it seems to be one of the more intense therapeutic grade essential oils. In 2009, researchers from the University of Oklahoma Health Sciences Center and Oklahoma City Veterans Affairs Medical Center published findings showing that frankincense oil can kill cells that cause cancer of the bladder. According to research published in the journal, *BMC Complementary and Alternative Medicine*, frankincense can potentially become a worthy alternative treatment for cancer of the bladder.

The oil also clears the lungs to help with breathing conditions such as asthma, bronchitis, and coughs; serves as a skin tonic to help rejuvenate aging skin; and minimizes skin inflammation, sores, and scars. All these benefits can also come from using frankincense in a blended massage oil or diluted in bath water, and in lotion.

In vapor therapy, which entails burning incense, frankincense oil is said to soothe and calm the mind and is popular for use in meditation and religious events. In religion, frankincense was and still is highly valued. For instance, the Catholic Church uses it during Mass and it is one of four main ingredients in Jewish ceremonial incense, an important part of the offerings of Sabbath.

Hyssop (*Hyssopus Officinalis*)

Hyssop is a perennial evergreen shrub that only grows 2 feet tall. A native of the Mediterranean area and now also cultivated in Europe, this shrub is woody with a hairy stem and miniscule lance-shaped green leaves and purplish-blue flowers. Hyssop oil is steam distilled from both the leaves and flowers. Four primary species of the hyssop shrub exist but aroma therapists concur that *hyssopus officinalis* is the best and main hyssop essential oil producer. France, Hungary, and Switzerland are now the main hyssop oil exporters.

Hyssop has been around since the biblical ages when it was used for its supposed cleansing properties for those suffering from leprosy and other ailments. Consider Psalms 51 7:10: "Purge me with hyssop, and I shall be clean: wash me, and I shall be whiter than snow." Although academics today debate about whether *hyssopus officinalis* is the same hyssop mentioned several times in the Bible and in other ancient writings, one constant remains: hyssop oil's benefits are clearly documented. Hippocrates, the father of modern medicine, is said to have prescribed hyssop oil for pleurisy, described as inflammation of the pleura membrane surrounding the lungs and usually characterized by painful breathing, coughing, as well as the buildup of fluid in the pleural cavity.

CHARACTERISTICS

Hyssop essential oil, classified as a base note, has a warm, sweet, and spicy aroma and ranges in color from colorless to pale yellowy-green. The oil is volatile, an attribute credited to its constituents like camphor and pinocamphone, both of which also contribute to its aroma.

BENEFITS AND USES

In aromatherapy, hyssop oil is favored for respiratory and digestive ailments. By rubbing it on affected areas, the oil treats bruises, colds, earaches, and sores. This oil is made from the hyssop flowers as an ingredient in syrups for coughs. Like many essential oils, you can also use hyssop in your bath water so it can impart some of its therapeutic qualities. The cosmetic industry uses hyssop oil in perfumes and the food and beverage industry uses it as a flavoring agent.

PRECAUTIONS

It is not recommended to use hyssop if you have a history of epilepsy or any seizure-related condition. Even those without this health history should not use, by ingestion or topical application, more than ten drops of hyssop oil per day.

Labdanum (*Cistus Ladanifer*)

Labdanum oil comes from a small, sticky shrub with lance-shaped white leaves that is native to the Middle East, the Mediterranean, Greece, and Spain but now is also cultivated in North America and other parts of the world. The oil is usually solvent extracted and is therefore not a true essential oil for aromatherapy purposes, even though it maintains some therapeutic properties.

It can also be steam distilled from the leaves and twigs of the labdanum shrub. Often called "rock rose" or "cistus oil," labdanum use dates back to several centuries ago when shepherds led goats and sheep through cistus shrubs so they could later collect the resin that would stick to the animals' furs. The resin was then sold to coastal traders, and they are believed to have ended up used for several purposes, including for the false beards Egyptian pharaohs wore. The resin is extracted by boiling leaves and twigs of the shrub and an absolute version is available by solvent extraction.

CHARACTERISTICS

Classified as a middle note, labdanum oil has a strong, musky aroma and like many resins it is viscously thick. Its constituents include camphene, limonene, borneol, and nerol, among many others. These give the oil its antiseptic, antimicrobial, astringent, and expectorant properties, making it useful in treating a variety of conditions.

BENEFITS AND USES

Past generations used labdanum to treat various conditions such as diarrhea, dysentery, ulcers, tumors, and skin ailments. It was also used to promote regular menstruation. Today, it can still be used for these conditions; however, like with any other essential oil, it should not replace proper medical advice and treatment. This essential oil can be found in soaps, lotions, massage oils, hair products, diffusers, air fresheners, bath oils, perfume, and laundry products.

Lime (*Citrus Aurantifolia*)

This essential oil comes from the fruits of a lime tree, which is considered a small tree because it only grows as tall as 15 feet. This wonderfully green tree, native to Asia but now widely cultivated, has sharp spines, smooth leaves, and small white flowers that vaguely resemble stars. Because the oil comes from a citrus fruit, it is best extracted from the fruit's peel by cold pressing. Steam distillation is also possible and is preferred by some aromatherapists. In steam distillation, whole ripe fruits are crushed to obtain the fresh citrus essence. Mexico has emerged as the leading exporter of therapeutic-grade lime oil used for aromatherapy because the oil is considered non-irritating, non-sensitizing, and non-phototoxic.

CHARACTERISTICS

If there ever was an essential oil that most of the world can guess its smell, it would be lime. Classified as a top note, lime essential oil has a sharp, citrus smell and like the fruit itself, the oil ranges in hue from pale yellow to light olive. It is viscously thin and like its relatives bergamot, grapefruit, and lemon, is laden with vitamin C, plus antiseptic, antibacterial, and antiviral properties.

BENEFITS AND USES

Chances are that you can find lime oil added to flavor or aroma a variety of food, household cleaning products, medicine, and beauty products. In aromatherapy, you can use it for bathing, massage, deodorizing, and vapor treatment. When you are battling a cold or sore throat, add two to three drops of lime oil to a steaming bowl of water, drape a towel over your head, and breathe in the invigorating essences for a few minutes for relief. You can also use the oil in a diffuser or vaporizer for a similar effect. Similarly 15 to 20 drops in your massage oil in dilution with about 1 ounce of sunflower oil will allow you to experience a relaxing massage that you will not soon forget.

Linden Blossom (*Tilia Cordata, Tilia Vulgaris*)

Extracted from parts of the linden tree, this oil is sometimes called lime blossom oil and can be easily confused with lime oil. The European native linden tree is medium to large sized with dark green heart-shaped leaves, green round fruits, and small yet fragrant yellowish-white flowers that bloom in late June or early July. The oil is extracted from these flowers.

CHARACTERISTICS

Linden blossom essential oil does not exist because the oil is a solvent extract, making the oil an absolute. The absolute version of the oil is also difficult to find.

It is classified as a top to medium note because of its strong citrus-like and floral aroma. The oil is of medium viscosity and has a deep brown color.

BENEFITS AND USES

When blended with equal parts jojoba oil, you can use it topically for fragrant, well nourished, and elastic skin. Therapeutically, linden blossom oil can be used as a sedative to decrease nervous tension, as an aid to minimize the symptoms brought on by colds and the flu, and as a muscle relaxant. Because of its fragrance, linden blossom is used in many products, including soap. It is also used in blending to enhance and complement bolder notes like woods and spices.

Litsea Cubeba (*May Chang*)

This uniquely named essential oil is steam distilled from the small, pepper-like fruits of the litsea cubeba, a native Chinese evergreen tree. It is a small tree that reaches 3 feet tall. Small quantities of this oil are also produced in Java, Indonesia, with the leaves rather than the fruits used for extraction.

CHARACTERISTICS

Because the oil is about 70 percent rich in citral, it has a fresh, intensely sweet, and lemony aroma. It is classified as a middle note, is yellow in color, and is viscously thin. In recent years, litsea cubeba has helped minimize the use of cheap synthetic citral made out of turpentine by the derivate industry that started because lemongrass, another citral-laden oil, became less available and thus more expensive. Both the Chinese litsea cubeba essential oil and the Indian lemongrass essential oil — its competition — are described by the industry as containing 75 percent citral.

BENEFITS AND USES

Litsea cubeba has been used to treat digestive disorders, nausea, aches, and pains like headaches. It can also be used in formulations to help combat acne, oily skin, asthma, and flatulence. It is very popular in the food, beverage, cosmetic, perfume, and fragrance industry because who can resist that lemony aroma or taste? In blending, litsea cubeba oil is also used to decrease the volatility of other citrus oils, providing an anchor to other citrus top notes that fade quickly. Blend it with other citrus oils or floral oils for a powerful therapeutic and fragrant blend.

Mandarin (*Citrus Reticulata*)

Mandarin oil is cold pressed from the easily peeled outer peel of the mandarin fruit, which comes from the glossy-leaved tree of the same name native to several Asian countries, including the Philippines, India, and China. It has long been esteemed for its medicinal properties in these countries.

Note that the terms "mandarin" and "tangerine" are sometimes interchanged as the fruits are two divergent varieties of easily peeled citrus. Tangerines are larger with more yellow skin than mandarins, which are deeply orange in color and have smooth skins.

CHARACTERISTICS

Unlike the deep orange colored mandarin fruit, mandarin oil has a light greenish-orange hue. Very much like the mandarin fruit, it has a strong, deeply sweet, citrus aroma. Classified as a top note, this oil has sedative properties that make it a handsome addition to any essential oil collection. Herbalists in France are known to recommend mandarin to help calm tension and irritability or to lull an excited child to sleep. Any parent with young children who has experienced a late night of endless bed jumping would benefit from using the oil in bath water or for a gentle massage.

Mandarin can be phototoxic so limit direct exposure to the sun while using it. Additionally, note that mandarin oil, like other cold pressed citrus oils, can deteriorate quickly, within six months, once it is exposed to air so store carefully.

USES AND BENEFITS

Mandarin is an affordable, gentle oil that can be used topically, even in children, to liven dull, acne prone, or scar-ridden skin. Use 2 teaspoons of mandarin oil blended with a drop of jasmine oil for such an application. It is hard to go wrong in blending mandarin oil, because it is very versatile and can blend with all other essential oils except those in the mint family, like catmint.

Marjoram (*Origanum Marjorana*)

This oil is steam distilled from the green oval leaves and pink flowers of a bushy perennial herb that is native to the Mediterranean region but is now cultivated around the world and even in the kitchen. Marjoram grows slowly and is less than 4 feet tall, but once it reaches maturity, it provides continuous harvest cycles.

CHARACTERISTICS

Marjoram oil has a warm, spicy aroma, ranges in color from pale yellow to amber, and is viscously thin. The oil's constituents include terpinolene and linalool, which likely contribute to its antiseptic, antiviral, diuretic, and sedative properties, making it a useful therapeutic grade essential oil.

BENEFITS AND USES

Marjoram has been used as a fragrant culinary herb for ages, but you can also use it in massage to relieve pain, stiffness, and soreness, especially those that are sports related or experienced during menstruation. Some aromatherapists recommend it as replacement for shaving creams and foam. Use it in a burner for a fragrant home or office.

Myrrh (*Commiphora Myrrha*)

As the age-old counterpart to the previously discussed frankincense, myrrh's history dates back thousands of years. Remember the biblical story of the Three

Wise Men bearing gifts? Myrrh and frankincense made up that list of gifts but that was not the first biblical mention for myrrh.

Myrrh is extracted from the sap of the *commiphora myrrha* tree, which belongs to the Burseraceae family, like frankincense's *boswellia thurifera* tree. An incision to the tree's bark releases a pale yellow gummy resin that is then left to dry into reddish-brown lumps from which the oil is steam distilled. Other myrrh botanical names are *commiphora molmol* and *balsamodendron myrrha*.

CHARACTERISTICS

Myrrh oil, which contains limonene among other constituents, is pale yellow and has a slightly spicy and woody smell that makes it a favorite to burn in incense. The oil is very viscous, especially when stored in a cool area, making it difficult to use when it is not in a blend, but it blends well with rose or jasmine.

BENEFITS AND USES

Myrrh oil is prized for its therapeutic qualities including as a digestive helper, wound healer, an astringent, anti-inflammatory, expectorant, stimulant, and antiviral. These qualities can be found in many products such as those used in oral hygiene, mouth sores, lotions, toiletries, and cough and cold medicines. A blend of myrrh in jojoba oil can do wonders for dull, cracked, dry, or aging skin. Myrrh oil is also said to promote healthy emotional and immune functions because of its effects on the body's cells and the limbic part of the brain that controls emotions.

Myrtle (*Myrtus Communis*)

Myrtle is the name of the essential oil steam distilled from the flowers, leaves, and sometimes stem of the myrtle, a large fragrant bush or small tree that is native to North Africa. Green myrtle is favored in aromatherapy because it is mild and works well as a respiratory treatment for conditions such as asthma.

The name, which comes from Greece, might have originated from Aphrodite, the Greek goddess of love and beauty who was worshipped with myrtle offerings in

• • •

the form of incense. Today, the Greek include myrtle in bridal bouquets, perhaps as a time honored reverence to Aphrodite.

CHARACTERISTICS

A middle note, myrtle oil has a fresh, herbal fragrance similar to that of eucalyptus oil. It is yellow to orange in color and viscously thin. Its components, including cineol and myrtenol, contribute to its therapeutic qualities such as antiseptic, deodorant, expectorant, and astringent. It also has a high alcohol content.

BENEFITS AND USES

Feel free to dab a drop of myrtle essential oil on each temple for quick relief for headaches. Try not to use more than a drop, because you may then end up feeling too euphoric.

The Greek physician Dioscorides is said to have favored macerated myrtle — myrtle leaves soaked in wine for a period of time — for lung and bladder infections. Although it is useful in treating urinary infections, today it is largely used for its antiseptic and astringent properties that help prevent and treat infections and oily or acne prone skin. Other sources recommend it as an aid to smoking cessation as it cleanses the body and helps curb cravings.

Nutmeg (*Myristica Fragrans*)

Nutmeg oil is steam distilled from the nutmeg seed produced from a native Sri Lankan and Indonesian evergreen tree that grows up to 65 feet tall and has dense foliage plus small yellow flowers. The worms eat the starch and fat found in the seeds, which are later crushed and dried in preparation for the steam distillation process. Nutmeg oil is also distilled in Europe, the United States, and other parts of the world from imported seeds but Indonesian and Sri Lankan oil is considered superior.

CHARACTERISTICS

Nutmeg oil, though non toxic, has a sharp, spicy aroma and could be dangerous for the eyes. The oil made from nutmeg husks is actually an ingredient in mace. The component myristicin is more plentiful in the husks, making them attractive for the weapon.

Nutmeg essential oil, though made from husk-less seeds, is still strong. It is a middle note, although some classify it as a top note. It is clear, viscously thin, and has numerous properties such as analgesic, antiseptic, carminative, digestive, laxative, stimulant, and tonic for the reproductive system, helping make menstruation regular and therefore increasing a woman's chances of getting pregnant.

BENEFITS AND USES

Nutmeg is a popular spice for those with culinary skills but in aromatherapy, nutmeg oil has been used in soap and candle making for its therapeutic purposes. Add four to six drops with 1 teaspoon of a carrier oil such as jojoba to your bath water and soak away sore muscles and relieve pain and poor circulation. A few drops in your massage oil will do the trick as well. You can also use it in a vaporizer, in a diffuser, or in a spray bottle mixed with 1 ounce of vodka to deodorize the air or to freshen linens and other household items.

PRECAUTIONS

Moderation is important when using this essential oil, because it can cause nausea and excessive heart rates when used in extreme quantities. It is not recommended for pregnant women, because it can cause premature contractions but can be used during labor to strengthen contractions and speed up the birth process.

Petitgrain (*Citrus uranium*)

Like neroli essential oil and orange essential oil, petitgrain essential oil comes from the orange tree. Petitgrain is now steam distilled from the leaves of the tree. It got its name "petit" meaning "little" in French, when it was extracted from

• • •

little, unripe "baby" fruits. Sources contend that the best petitgrain essential oil comes from the steam distillation of the twigs and buds. The tree is native to the Mediterranean region and cheaper grades are imported from the South American country of Paraguay.

CHARACTERISTICS

Petitgrain essential oil is a top note oil with a woody, slightly floral aroma and a pale yellow to amber hue. It is viscously thin but is an uplifting oil that can easily reduce the kind of mental fatigue associated with stress and anxiety.

BENEFITS AND USES

Petitgrain oil acts wonderfully in a diffuser to relieve mental fatigue and stress; it is like having tiny little hands massage stress from your whole body. It also promotes sleep by chasing away insomnia. Use it in a blend with neroli for an inspiring massage or add it to your lotion. Other uses include as an ingredient in the perfume industry's eau-de-cologne and as an anti-infectious, antibacterial, and digestive tonic.

Pine (*Pinus Sylvestris*)

Pine essential oil holds the distinction of coming from one of the most widely recognized trees in the world. The pine tree, sometimes called Scotch pine, is a 130-foot tall conifer-shaped evergreen tree with needle-like green leaves, pointy brown cones, yellow flowers, and reddish-brown fissured or cracked bark. The essential oil is extracted by steam distilling the flower buds, twigs, and needle-like leaves.

Several different species of pine are used to extract the essential oil and they are often labeled as "pine oil," a fact that can easily confuse a novice who is not familiar with each botanical name. *Pinus sylvestris* is the most therapeutic and safe pine oil, while others such as *pinus mugo* and *pinus palustris*, the longleaf pine, are less therapeutic and highly irritating to the skin. They are best used for raw materials for products such as turpentine.

CHARACTERISTICS

If you can imagine being in a forest during Christmas surrounded by nothing but the smell of a freshly cut Christmas tree, then you know the refreshing aroma of pine oil. It has a watery viscosity, is generally pale yellow, and is classified as a middle note.

BENEFITS AND USES

Use it in a diffuser, vaporizer, or blended with cedarwood oil for massage to ease asthma, colds, sinus infections, muscle aches, and hangovers. You can also use it in saunas and steam baths for similar benefits and as an alternative to harsh pharmaceutical concoctions.

Herbalists recommend it to relieve all sorts of fatigue including those of the physical, mental, and sexual nature. It can also be used to treat sores, cuts, scabies, lice, excessive perspiration, rheumatism, arthritis, gout, as well as asthma, bronchitis, coughs, colds, and sinusitis.

Roman Chamomile (*Chamaemelum Nobile*)

This essential oil is steam distilled from the flower heads of a perennial herb that is native to Southern and Western Europe but now cultivated in the United States and other parts of the world. The herb has feathery pinnated leaves, which hang in pairs on opposite sides of the stem, and white flowers that are reminiscent of daisies but larger than those from the German chamomile herb. Roman chamomile is only one of four species of chamomile native to Britain with therapeutic properties. This allows the market to be flooded with low-grade oils, making it useful to have a keen eye and nose when looking to purchase this oil.

CHARACTERISTICS

This middle note oil has an herbaceous, warm, sweet, and fruity aroma. It is of medium viscosity and has a natural blue hue like German chamomile thanks to the component azulene. Roman chamomile's therapeutic properties include being a sedative, antiseptic, and anti-inflammatory.

BENEFITS AND USES

Roman chamomile essential oil is listed in the *British Herbal Pharmacopoeia,* a publication that promotes the responsible use of herbal medicines, for treatment of anorexia, nausea, morning sickness, and flatulent dyspepsia (acid indigestion) associated with mental stress. In aromatherapy, Roman chamomile is used to counter insomnia and it makes good tea that is useful in relaxing the drinker.

Spruce (*Picea Mariana*)

Spruce essential oil is steam distilled from the needles and twigs of the spruce tree, a Canadian native. It is found in wet swamp areas and is sometimes called black spruce.

CHARACTERISTICS

It has a fresh, pleasant, and woody middle note aroma that is both calming and elevating. It is viscously thin, has a clear to pale yellow hue, and contains limonene, among other components.

BENEFITS AND USES

Spruce essential oil has long been used in massage, saunas, steam baths, and baths to relieve soreness and open up blocked pores. The oil can also be used topically in dilution, blends, or in lotions; as a dietary supplement if you add a drop in rice milk; or in a deodorizer for aroma. Spruce essential oil is recommended for muscle aches, painful joints, poor circulation, strains, and sprains. One source recommends a blend of spruce oil and helichrysum — an oil known for its toning properties — to help soothe injuries to ligaments, muscles, and tendons while speeding up healing and preventing the formation of often ugly scars.

Thyme (*Thymus Vulgaris*)

This highly potent essential oil is steam distilled from the flowering tops and leaves of an evergreen shrub that only grows to about 20 inches tall. The shrub has small, elliptical greenish-gray leaves and pale purple or white flowers.

CHARACTERISTICS

Thyme essential oil has a fresh, medicinal, and herbaceous aroma. This plant has, among other properties, strong antiseptic qualities that can actually become toxic if used improperly. Thyme oil is classified as a middle note and has medium viscosity.

BENEFITS AND USES

Because the Greek word "thymos" means "to perfume," it is hardly a surprise that thyme oil is used in perfumery. In aromatherapy, thyme oil treats dandruff and other scalp issues, hair loss, and carbuncles, those nasty two-headed boils.

It has also been useful for those suffering from respiratory illnesses such as asthma, bronchitis, coughs, and colds by removing phlegm and mucus from the chest and throat. It is also useful in countering arthritis, gout, and rheumatism. You will find its component, thymol, listed as an ingredient in mouthwash, because it can kill the microorganisms causing gingivitis and plaque.

Even some conventional doctors have had to contend with thyme's potency, which has been found to be fatal to a number of bacterium including anthrax bacillus, typhoid bacillus, as well as tuberculosis salmonella and staphylococcus. Thyme oil can also be a digestive stimulant that can help ease dyspepsia, reduce gastric infections, and reduce flatulence.

Yarrow (*Achillea Millefolium*)

Yarrow oil comes from a native Bulgarian perennial herb that grows to a height of up to 3 feet and has feathery, fern-like leaves and pinkish-white flower heads. Yarrow is also known as milfoil or common yarrow.

• • •

CHARACTERISTICS

Yarrow oil is laden with chamazulene and azulene, which gives it a vivid, dark blue hue. It is classified as a middle note and has a sweet, warm, and herbal aroma coupled with a watery viscosity.

BENEFITS AND USES

Yarrow oil has many therapeutic benefits such as improving circulatory disorders like varicose veins and hemorrhoids. It can also help regulate menstruation, menopause-related problems, digestive-related problems like flatulence and constipation, and can be used in the nervous system to counter stress and insomnia. By churning up a 3:1 salve of yarrow oil and beeswax, you can create a highly beneficial concoction for the skin that can help heal and decrease the appearance of inflamed skin, eczema, rashes, wounds, cuts, scars, and burns.

With the knowledge of essential oils, their characteristics, benefits, and uses, comes the need to know how to properly use the oils. It is important to know how to blend two or more oils together to produce powerful, multi-use and multi-benefit products. *The next chapter will contain some tips on how you can blend essential oils.*

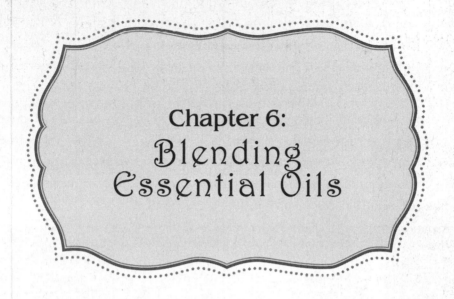

Chapter 6:
Blending Essential Oils

There really is no right or wrong way to create an essential oil aromatherapy blend. Once you have educated yourself on each oil you desire for your blend, you will be well on your way to creating a therapeutic concoction that can be appreciated not only by yourself, but by others.

Looking at the Notes

Much like the notes of a piano signify high or low pitch, essential oil notes signify the strength and longevity of an aroma. Why is it that you are able to smell some perfumes long after the wearer has left a room or building? This is because some essential oils used in the perfumes are more volatile and evaporate faster, while others linger for hours. Classifying oils into notes is not an exact science and it tends to be very subjective, but here are some easily remembered tips.

There are three note categories used to classify essential oils: Top, middle, and base. Fast evaporating oils — the wearer comes in smelling fragrantly, the smell lasts for one or two hours, and then stops smelling fragrantly — are called **top**

• • •

notes. On the other hand, when the scent lasts for two to four hours and still smells fragrantly, this is most likely a **middle note** scent. When the perfume wearer leaves your presence but the scent lingers for even a day afterwards, he or she is most definitely wearing a **base note**.

It is not unusual to find some essential oils listed in two or more of these categories, especially when they are used in blends. Top notes blended with base notes may very well become middle notes as base oils act as anchors, preventing fast evaporation. Refer to the following table for classifications of the previously discussed essential oils. Each oil is listed where it best fits.

Top Notes	Middle Notes		Base Notes
• Allspice	• Angelica root	• Myrtle	• Balsam of Peru
• Anise	• Bay	• Neroli	• Cananga
• Anise, star	• Black pepper	• Nutmeg	• Cedarwood
• Basil	• Cardamom	• Pine	• Cumin
• Bergamot	• Carrot seed	• Roman chamomile	• Frankincense
• Cinnamon bark	• Catmint		• Ginger
• Citronella	• Chamomile	• Rose	• Jasmine
• Eucalyptus	• Clary sage	• Rose geranium	• Labdanum
• Grapefruit	• Clove	• Rosemary	• Myrrh
• Hyssop	• Coriander	• Rosewood	• Patchouli
• Lavender	• Cypress	• Spruce	• Sandalwood
• Lemon	• Dill	• Tea tree	• Vanilla
• Lemongrass	• Fennel	• Thyme	• Ylang-ylang
• Lime	• Fir	• Yarrow	
• Mandarin	• Juniper		
• Orange, sweet	• Linden blossom		
• Peppermint	• Litsea cubeba		
• Petitgrain	• Marjoram		

Aromatic Blends

Whether you are an experienced aromatherapy professional or a novice, you have the power to create aromatic blends that are wonderfully therapeutic and sensationally smelling, which after all is the main purpose of aromatherapy. You can create blends of two or more essential oils in carrier oils for natural skin care — lotions, facial masks, bath and massage oils — home recipes like deodorizers, stain removers, and for therapeutic reasons to treat common conditions. In order to stay within the confines of natural body care, take care to use only the best, most natural ingredients such as essential oils, carrier oils, and water that you can afford.

Before creating these blends, you should first educate yourself on each essential oil you desire to use. Feel free to become a mad scientist, but even a mad scientist would not want to go into a chemical lab and experiment with mixing sometimes toxic or explosive chemicals without really knowing the full potential of the damage that can occur in the process.

It is worthy to note that there are about seven types of essential oil aroma categories: citrus, earthy, floral, herbal, minty, spicy, and woody. There is an additional category covering camphorous — medicinal — oils such as eucalyptus and tea tree. Oils in the same category usually blend well together but a few exceptions do exist and they will be addressed as each category is further explained. Also note that oils from different categories can blend well together.

Citrus

A good citrus blend will have you feeling like you just walked into a room at the very same time an orange was being peeled. The aroma no doubt conjures up images of summer, laughter, and youthfulness. Citrus essential oils include orange, lemon, and lime and are usually top notes that brighten up blends and the users of those blends. They blend well together and blend well with spicy and floral notes, with the exception of the highly floral neroli oil, which can result in a heady, overpowering blend.

Earthy

Think of the smell of rain as it hits the forest ground on a warm afternoon. Earthy blends like patchouli and helichrysum are base notes that blend well with each other and with minty oils like peppermint. As with many essential oil blends, use your nose to guide you during the blending process, only avoiding blends that do not appeal to your sense of smell.

Floral

By now you know that the unmistakable scent and properties of roses are as equally good on the skin as they are for general well being. These oils can be either top, middle, and base notes and include rose, rose geranium, juniper, lavender, and neroli and can be used together and in carrier oil for an uplifting and relaxing aroma. They also blend well with spicy, citrus, and woody oils.

Herbal

Basil and rosemary are two examples of herbal essential oils, which, like their name suggests, smell like herbs that can be found in your kitchen cabinet. They can be of either top, middle, or base notes and they blend well with each other and with minty oils.

Minty

Catmint, peppermint, and spearmint belong in this herb category. They are wonderfully refreshing and aromatic oils of top and middle note classifications that make you think of freshness, and especially, fresh breath. They blend well with woody and herbal oils, but they also blend well with some floral oils like lavender and some citrus oils like lemon.

Spicy

The spicy category of herbs has allspice, cinnamon, clove, and nutmeg, which are top, middle, and base notes that blend well with each other and also with floral and citrus oils. Try not to overpower your blend with more than two varieties of spicy oils. For example, using nutmeg oil in a blend with ginger oil is sufficient, not just for therapeutic reasons, but if you are fond of the holiday season, it can remind you of just how enjoyable that time of year can be.

Woody

Oils in this category can be top, middle, or base note classifications with aromas that are reminiscent of fresh sawdust with a hint of balsamic. They are versatile when it comes to blending, because they can blend well with all other essential oil categories for maximum therapeutic effects. Woody oils include carrot seed, cedarwood, and pine.

Therapeutic Blends

The word "therapeutic" describes the action of healing diseases and other afflictions humans suffer. When essential oils are administered for these reasons, they are said to be therapeutic. In aromatherapy, creating blends has multiple purposes that combine exceptional smell with therapeutic benefits for both the mind and the body. Blends should always be created for maximum therapeutic effects and their composition should depend on their intended use.

For example, a vanilla and sandalwood blend would make a balanced and sweet-smelling perfume that many women can appreciate. A blend of carrot seed essential oil, helichrysum, roman chamomile, rose geranium, and ylang-ylang in a hazelnut carrier oil base would create a powerful lotion blend to protect the skin against sun damage, minimize the appearance of scars, and delay the formation of wrinkles. Blending geranium, myrtle, sage, and spearmint in a diffuser or for massage can benefit the endocrine system, which works to secrete hormones directly into the blood, to give you high energy on a dragging day.

Substituting Different Essential Oils

There are times when you might have to substitute one or more essential oils in a blend because you are either sensitive or allergic to the oil, the aroma does not inspire you, availability is limited, or it is too expensive. Whatever the reason, your blend will do much better, especially therapeutically, if you select substitutions that belong to the same group. Examples of these substitutions, which can go both ways, are peppermint for spearmint, clove for cinnamon, sweet orange for mandarin, and lemon for grapefruit.

Practical Tips When Blending Oils

The most important things to remember when blending oils are safety, following your intuition, and respecting your sense of smell. Follow the safety tips discussed in Chapter 1 when dealing with essential oils. To create a captivating aromatic blend, consider aging your oils for at least a week before blending them and after blending them. Your nose will tell you when your blend is ready or when you should avoid creating the blend that way again.

Try to blend on a small scale. It would not be prudent to invest in costly oils and then blend multiple oils together before discovering that you completely hate the blend you created. Try using bottles that have dropper tops, keeping in mind that viscous oils such as vanilla oleoresin and benzoin flow through droppers best once they have been diluted. But if you are missing droppers, you can still blend your oils in a clean, ideally sterile, kitchen gadget like a tablespoon.

Although essential oils are natural, they are not without some grave dangers. There are essential oils that are considered dangerous and even toxic for human and animal consumption and are therefore best to avoid, especially by novices.

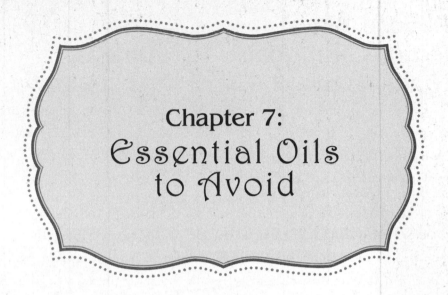

Chapter 7: Essential Oils to Avoid

This is a group of more than 30 oils that you should keep at arms length, especially if you are not a trained aromatherapy professional, because they can be toxic. The plants these oils are extracted from tend to have other non-toxic uses that we will examine.

Ajowan (*Trachyspermum Ammi*)

Ajowan essential oil is steam distilled from the seed of the *trachyspermum ammi* herb that belongs to the umbelliferae family, which also includes dill and cumin, and is used frequently in Indian cooking. Only by cooking this oil can you destroy the toxic oils found within it. The herb is also called bishop's weed or carom and is found in India, Egypt, and the West Indies.

Ajowan has high levels of thymol that makes it a strong antiseptic, germicide, and stimulant, useful in Ayurvedic medicine to treat cholera and for other conditions. But thymol is also the component that should be avoided, because it can be toxic in high levels. The cosmetics industry extracts thymol from the oil and uses it as an ingredient in mouthwash and in body soaps under the name "thymene."

Almond, Bitter (*Prunus Amygdalus Var. Amara*)

This oil, not be confused with the carrier oil sweet almond, is steam distilled from the bitter almond tree that is native to Africa and Asia but is now found in Egypt, Morocco, Tunisia, and Turkey. The oil comes from separating almond kernels from their shells before crushing them in a press and then macerating the resulting powder in water for steam distillation.

Bitter almond essential oil is not recommended for use in therapy because it contains prussic acid, also known as cyanide, a well known poison. The food industry uses bitter almond essence for food flavoring, but only after the prussic acid is removed from the almond kernels by a refining process that includes washing it in alkaline solutions.

Arborvitae (*Thuja Occidentalis*)

This tree, sometimes called cedar leaf or yellow cedar, is grown in Canada and Europe. It has a conical shape and can grow up to 30 feet tall. The name thuja is said to be the Latin form of the Greek word "thuo" that means "to sacrifice." The trees are valuable as hedge trees but are not recommended for herbal use. The oil distilled from leaves and twigs is an irritant that contains pinipicrin and tannic acid, both powerful toxins that can quickly render an average-sized person unconscious and spastic after only 15 drops of usage. If ingested, it also causes stomach irritation and distension whereby the stomach swells on the outside because of excessive air.

Arnica (*Arnica Montana*)

Arnica essential oil is extracted from the dried daisy-like flower heads and roots of a perennial plant also known as "wolf's bane" or "leopard's bane" that is native to Siberia and the mountainous parts of Europe. The oil has a long history of use in homeopathic medicine for wound healing, among other uses, dating back hundreds of years.

Although the oil is quite powerful in therapy for heart conditions such as angina, coronary artery disease, for wounds, and as a pain reliever, it contains arnicin, a bitter and toxic yellow crystalline. Arnica essential oil is diluted heavily when used in commercially available topical creams and ointments. It is also used as a tincture for compresses and poultices. **Poultices** are moist preparations made out of the herb's flowers macerated (soaked) in alcohol for at least a week. They are used to relieve bruises, sprains, inflammation, and soreness.

Birch, Sweet (*Betula Lenta*)

Sweet birch essential oil is extracted from a tree grown in parts of the United States such as New York, New Hampshire, and Vermont. The tree is also known as black birch or cherry birch, and bears unique wood that, when exposed to air, darkens to a color that resembles mahogany and is used for furniture. The oil contains methyl salicylate, which is now used as a food flavor and in medicine, but it can be fatally poisonous if ingested and highly irritating on the skin if handled by an untrained aromatherapist.

Boldo Leaf (*Peumus Boldus*)

Boldo leaf essential oil is distilled from the slow-growing peumus boldus, also known as boldu, boldea, or boldoa that is native to South America and has been used to treat liver, gallbladder, and urinary problems. The oil has anti-inflammatory, antioxidant, diuretic, and sedative properties but at the same time, it can cause a user's blood to thin dangerously and cause birth defects in pregnant women.

Broom, Spanish (*Spartium Junceum*)

Spanish broom absolute oil is solvent extracted from the flowers of the weed-like deciduous plant of the same name that is native to the Mediterranean area. It is used as an ornamental ground cover; its fibers are used for weaving and making paper; and its yellow flowers are used to make a yellow dye. The oil is used in perfumery around the world but is highly upsetting to the stomach if ingested and irritating to the skin if used topically.

Calamus (*Acorus Calamus*)

Calamus essential oil is steam distilled from the root of *acorus calamus* whose properties vary according to the plant's geographic location. European- and Asian-grown calamus have high levels of asarone, a compound that can be toxic to the skin, is considered a carcinogenic, and is also known to cause hallucination and chromosome damage. Versions of the plant cultivated in North America do not have asarone and are considered safe to use when diluted.

Camphor (*Cinnamomum Camphora*)

Camphor essential oil is steam distilled from the roots, wood, and branches of *cinnamomum camphora*, a native Taiwanese tree also known as *laurus camphora*, hon-sho, or gum camphor. The oil, though therapeutic if used with care, contains the toxic and carcinogenic safrole.

Cassia (*Cinnamomum Cassia*)

The oil is extracted from the thick, leathery leaves, twigs, and bark of *laurus cassia*, which is native to China and is closely related to *laurus camphora*, the tree that produces camphor essential oil. This tree does not grow quite as tall as its relative; it reaches just 65 feet tall and has thick, leathery leaves and small white flowers. The tree's bark is used to flavor foods like curry, candies, and soft drinks and the oil is highly therapeutic if used in vaporizers and in diffusers. Avoid using on the skin to prevent irritation.

Common Wormwood (*Artemisia Vulgaris*)

The oil comes from a perennial herb that can grow almost 6 feet tall and tends to thrive in poor, hot, alkaline soil. The plant was once used in the kitchen to stuff fatty meats and to treat a variety of problems such as eczema and psoriasis, but the oil contains alpha-thujone, a compound considered to be toxic.

Deertongue (*Trisilia Odoratissima*)

Deertongue oil is solvent extracted from the tongue-shaped leaves of an herb characterized by a long and narrow reddish-purplish streak at the base. The plant, trisilia odoratissima, is also known as vanilla leaf or wild vanilla because the leaves emanate a distinctive vanilla aroma when crushed, due to a naturally-occurring component called coumarin.

Coumarin is therapeutically useful as a blood thinner and anti-fungal; however, it should not be used when taking anticoagulants because it can dangerously increase blood flow in the veins. Additionally, studies have found that even small amounts of coumarin can cause liver damage in sensitive people. Thankfully, the damage is not permanent and can be reversed when usage stops.

Garlic (*Allium Sativum*)

Garlic essential oil is extracted from a perennial bulbous plant now cultivated widely but indigenous to Sibera. The bulb part of the plant is known and used widely in cooking. Garlic oil, though considered non toxic and non irritant, has been known to cause botulism, a major stomach illness that can lead to death and is attributed to garlic's sulphurous nature. Botulism is caused by the bacterium *clostridium botulinum* and occurs easily when the oil is stored improperly, at room temperature. Remember that refrigerating oils not only helps them last longer, it is also a good way to keep away harmful organisms like bacteria.

Horseradish (*Armoracia Rusticana*)

Horseradish essential oil is steam or water distilled from the water-logged roots of the *armoracia rusticana* perennial plant that belongs to the Brassicaceae family, which includes cabbages. The plant is believed to be native to southeastern Europe and parts of Asia, but today it is cultivated around the world. The plant's roots are edible, but its leaves are used either as a vegetable or ground for use as a condiment.

Horseradish oil is not recommended for ingestion because it contains allyl isothiocyanate, a component that forms when the plant's roots are cut, allowing existing enzymes to break down and produce allyl isothiocyanate, which is highly irritating to skin, eyes, nose, and sinuses.

Jaborandi (*Pilocarpus Jaborandi*)

The leaves of the shrubby jaborandi tree, native to the West Indies as well as Central and South America, contain the jaborandi essential oil. In South America, herbalists use jaborandi to treat asthma, tonsillitis, catarrh — excessive mucus buildup in the nose and throat — rheumatism, and nausea. It is considered a toxic oil because it contains the compound pilocarpine, which is known to cause vision disturbances, vomiting, diarrhea, and respiratory distress that can result in cardiac collapse. The presence of tyramine in the oil can also cause hypertension.

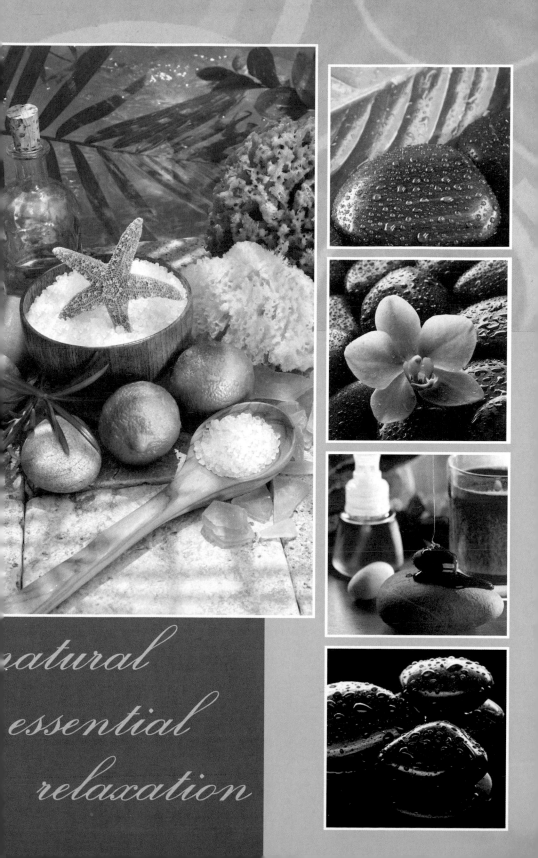

natural

essential

relaxation

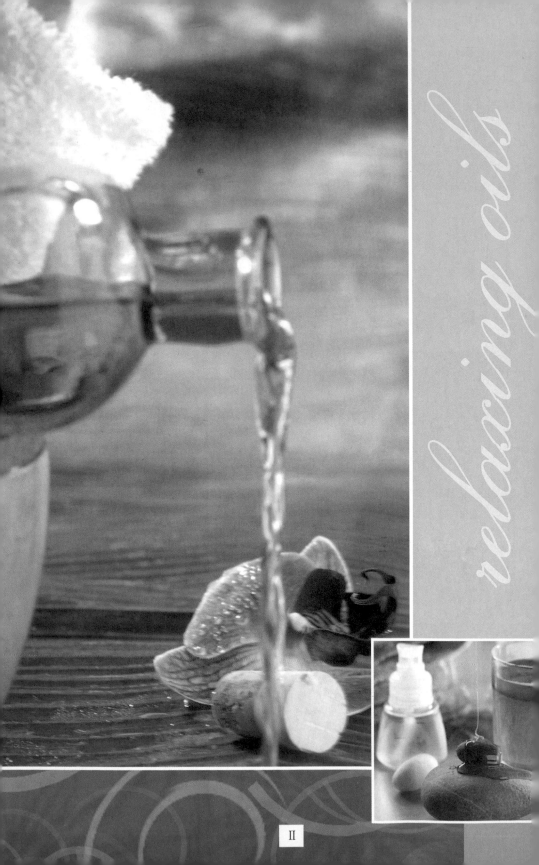

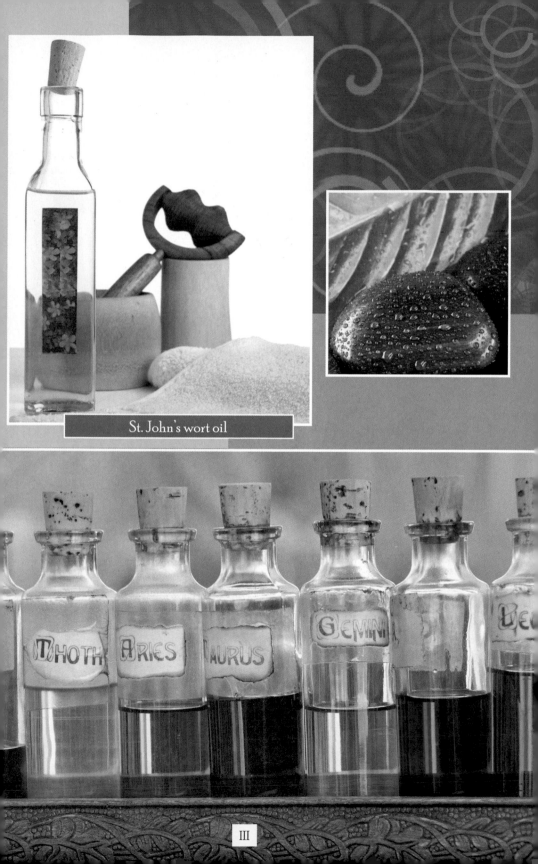

St. John's wort oil

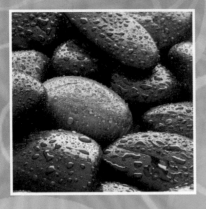

Massage oils

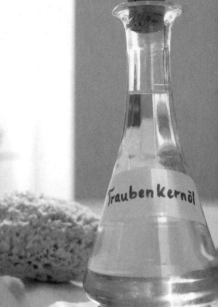

Grapeseed oil and a natural sponge

IV

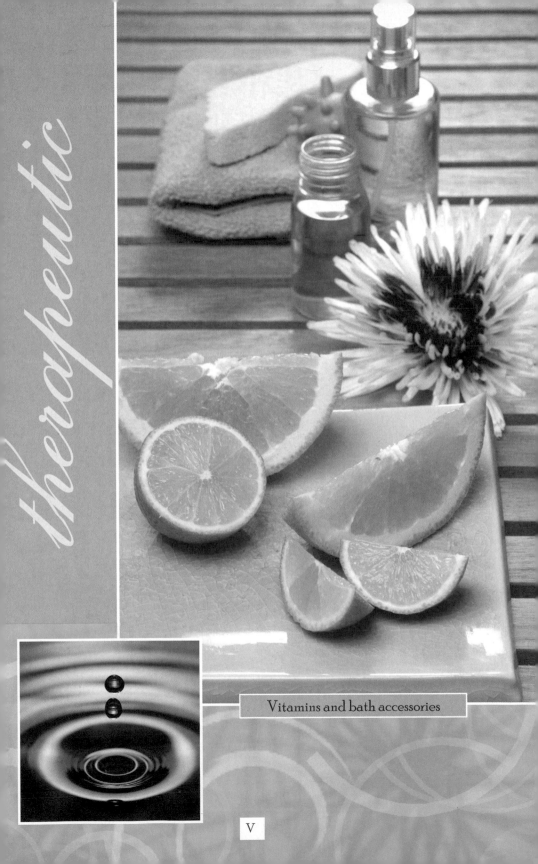

therapeutic

Vitamins and bath accessories

V

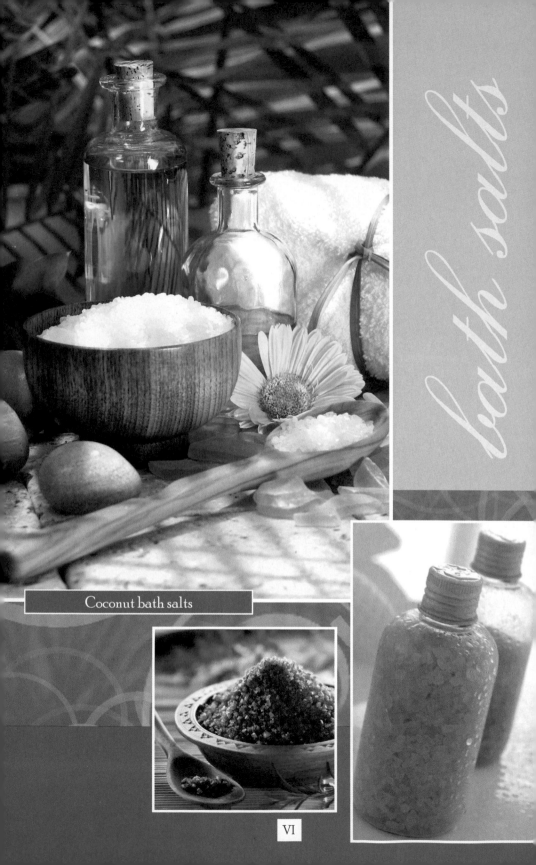

bath salts

Coconut bath salts

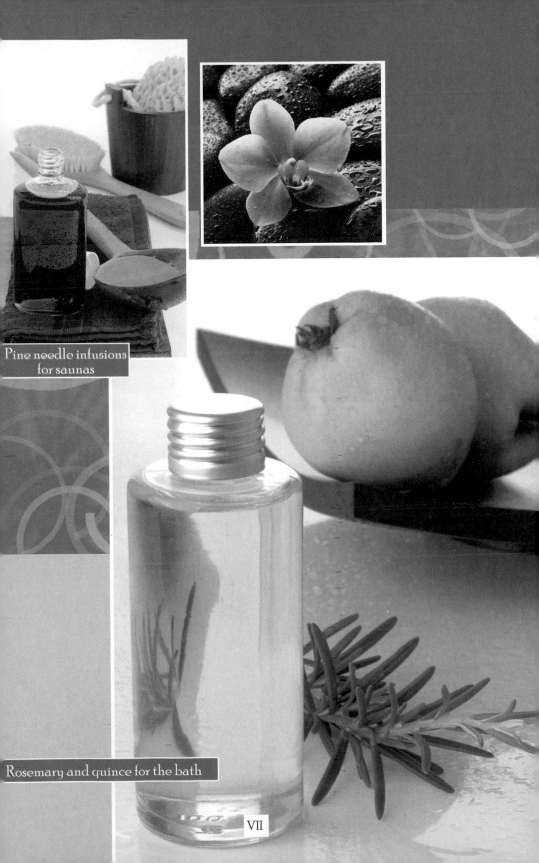

Pine needle infusions for saunas

Rosemary and quince for the bath

VII

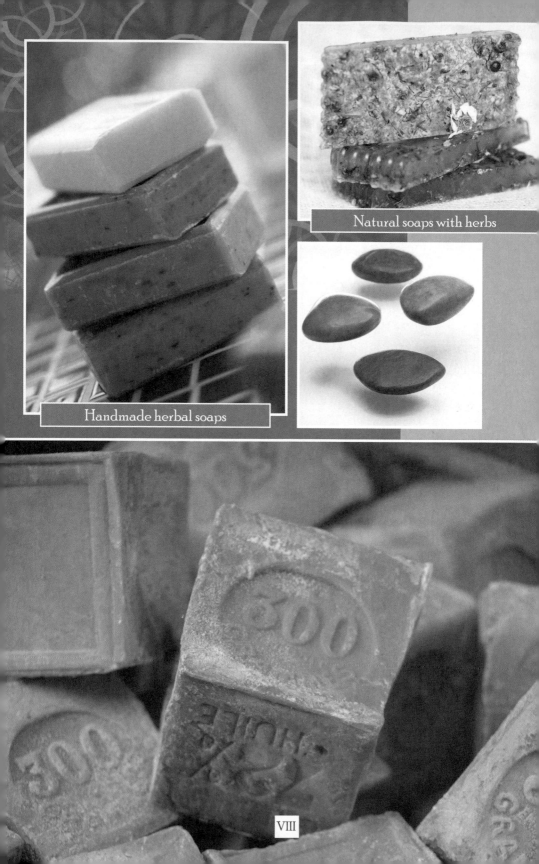

Natural soaps with herbs

Handmade herbal soaps

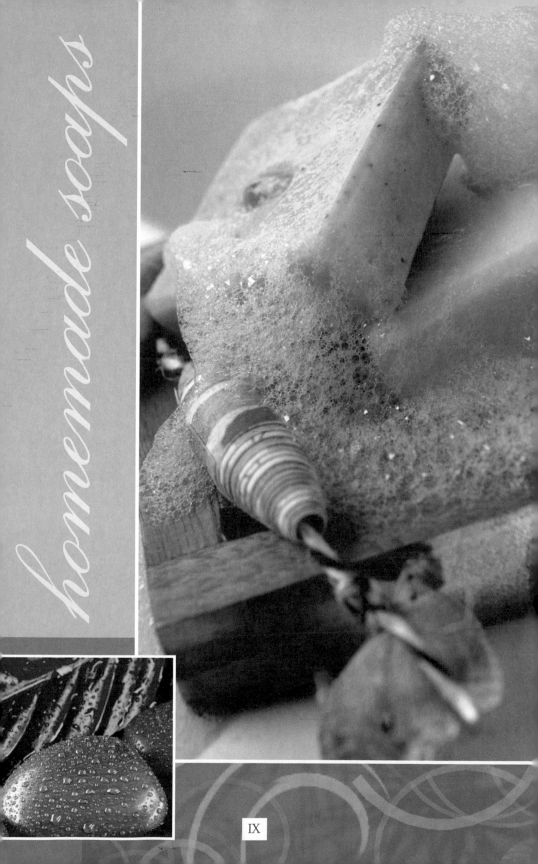

homemade soaps

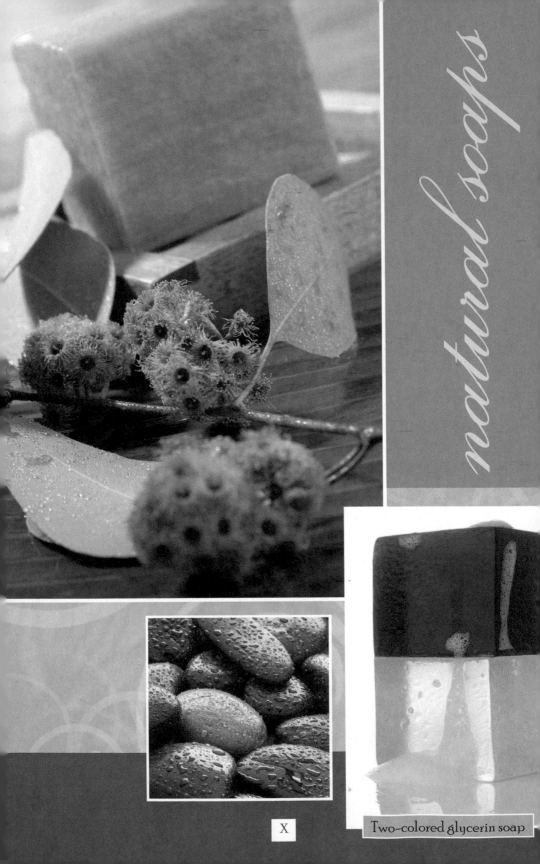

natural soaps

Two-colored glycerin soap

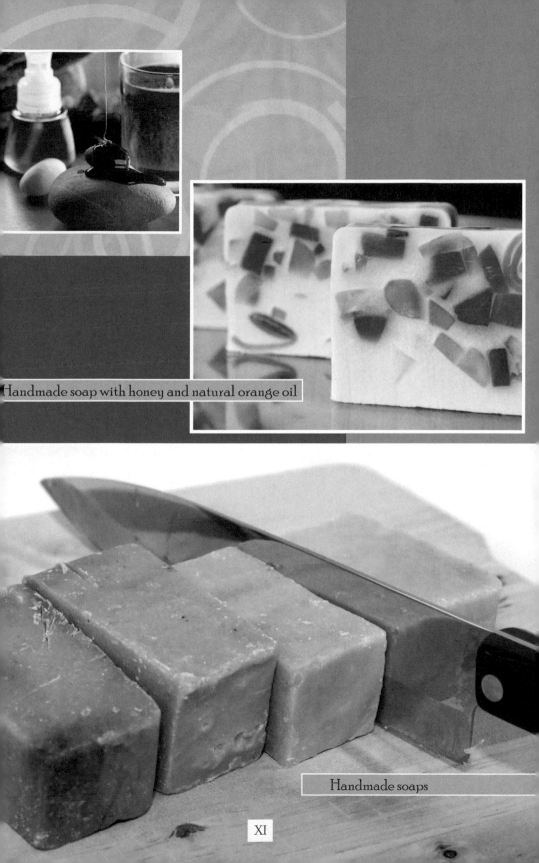

Handmade soap with honey and natural orange oil

Handmade soaps

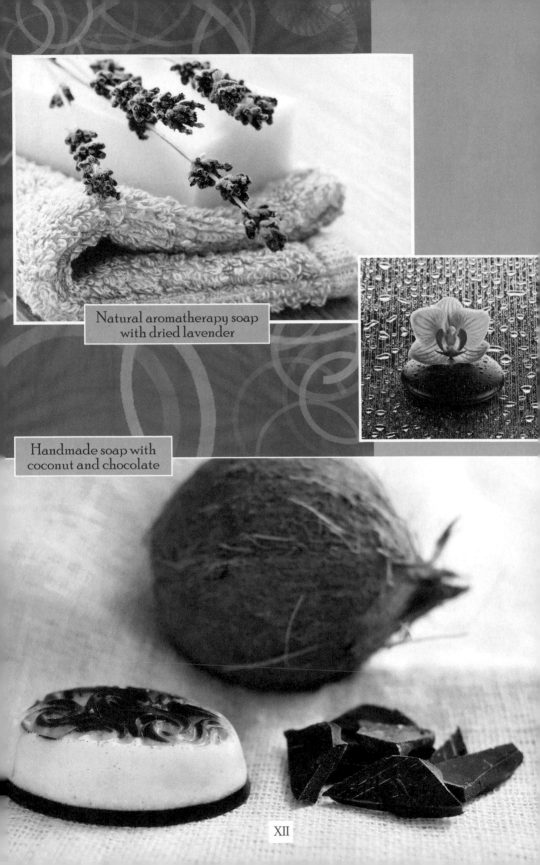

Natural aromatherapy soap
with dried lavender

Handmade soap with
coconut and chocolate

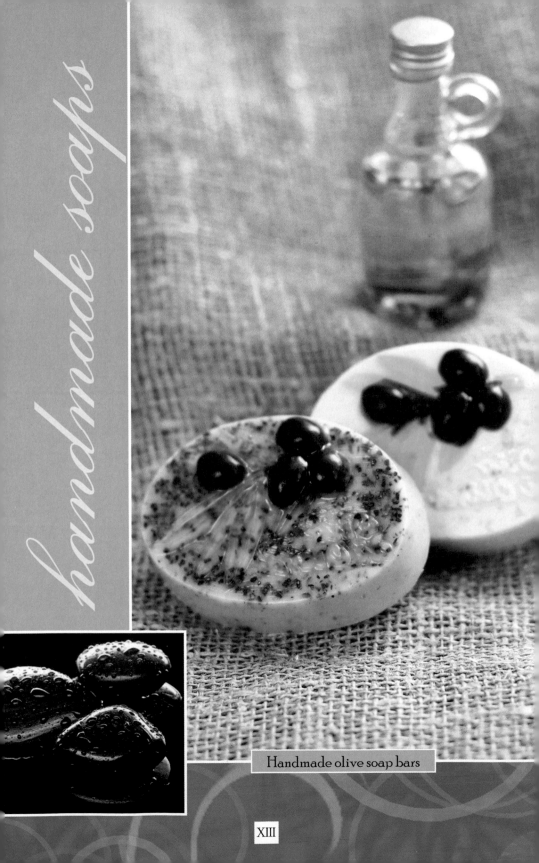

handmade soaps

Handmade olive soap bars

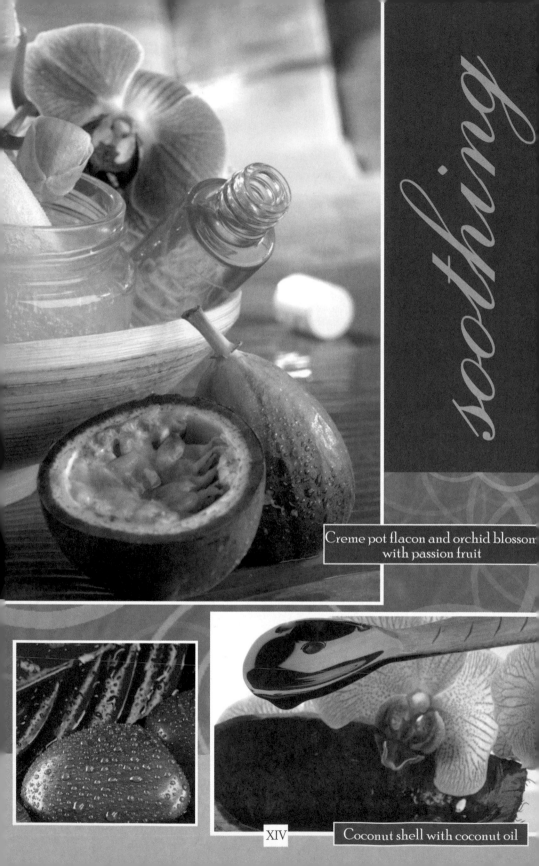

soothing

Creme pot flacon and orchid blossom
with passion fruit

Coconut shell with coconut oil

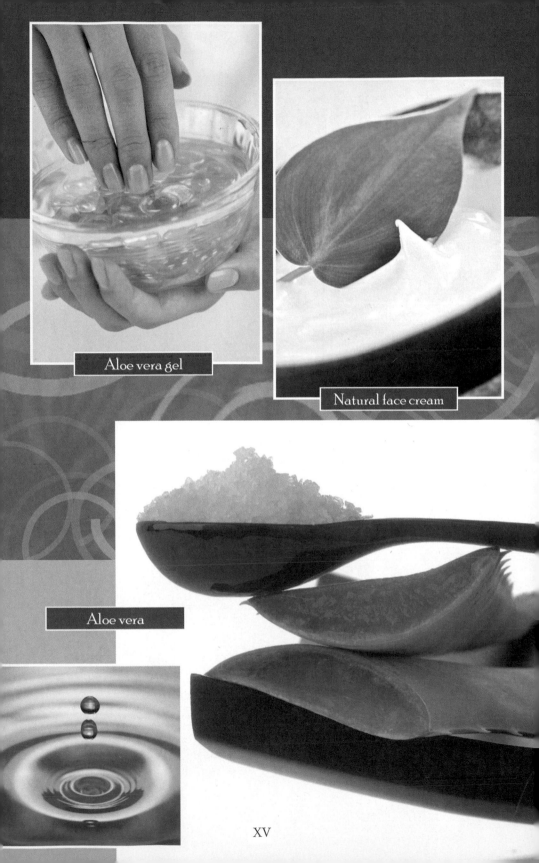

Aloe vera gel

Natural face cream

Aloe vera

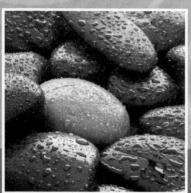

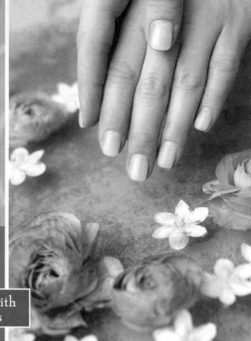

Aromatherapy session with flowers, water, and oils

Preparing an aromatherapy session

Lavender Cotton (*Santolina Chamaecyparissus*)

Lavender cotton is a hardy ornamental evergreen herb that thrives in extreme conditions, including below freezing temperatures, and grows about 2 feet tall. It has gray foliage and small yellow flowers. The plant's foliage can be packaged in sachets or hung in bunches to repel moths, and the flowers can be used as everlasting ornamentals. The essential oil of lavender cotton is distilled from the whole plant, and it is not recommended in therapy because it is toxic.

Mustard, Black (*Brassica Nigra*)

Mustard oil, as do mustard seeds, comes from *brassica nigra*, an annual plant characterized by a branched stem, U-shaped leaves about 6 inches long, and bright yellow flowers. Mustard seeds have long been used in herbal medicine to promote appetite, help with digestion, coughs and colds, arthritis, and other pains. The oil, on the other hand, contains allyl isothiocyanate, formed when mustard seeds come in contact with water. The level of allyl isothiocyanate in mustard oil is said to be more than 90 percent, making it very toxic and very irritating to the skin and mucus membranes.

Onion (*Allium Cepa*)

Onion oil is steam distilled from the widely-used onion bulb originally cultivated in the Middle East and Asia but now available worldwide and mostly used for culinary purposes. Onion oil is seldom used in aromatherapy products mainly because some consider its aroma offensive, but its irritant properties, which are evident each time you cut an onion, certainly contribute to why it is on this list of uncommon oils. The oil can be found in some pharmaceutical blends to treat coughs and colds.

Oregano (*Origanum Vulgare*)

Oregano oil is one of the most potent essential oils you can find. In the Mediterranean area, it is mostly steam distilled from the leaves of *origanum vulgare* and used for a variety of reasons related to its anti-bacterial, anti-fungal, and anti-oxidant properties. One of the reasons it is used is for its abilities to slow down food spoilage. Because of oregano oil's potency, it has the potential to be very irritating to the skin.

Orris Root (*Iris Florentina, Iris Pallida*)

The iris plants that carry orrisroot oil in their roots are native to Europe and are known for their beautiful yellow-white blooms and their ability to adapt to most temperate conditions. For ancient Europeans, the plant was used in scepters as a symbol of power and majesty. In Florence, Italy, the plant's roots, which resemble ginger, are sold as "ghiaggiuolo" and can be chewed for the same effect as toothpaste. Powdered orris root can be used as a snuff to alleviate sinus headaches and orris root oil works well in perfumes. The oil contains the compound iridin, which is known to be poisonous in humans and animals.

Pennyroyal (*Mentha Pulegium*)

Pennyroyal is a perennial herb native to Europe that grows up to 20 inches tall and has smooth, round stalks, gray-green oval leaves, lilac flowers, and a fibrous creeping root. The leaves carry the essential oil that is mostly extracted by steam distillation. The herb has been found useful in treating a variety of complaints, such as those related to menstruation. The oil, however, is toxic and even in small quantities can cause liver and lung damage.

Rue (*Ruta Graveolens*)

This oil has the distinction of being distilled from an herb considered by some to be the most bitter herb in the world. The age-old herb mentioned in the Bible has woody branches, small, smooth blue-green leaves, and small yellowish-green flowers. It has been used as a homeopathic herb to alleviate varicose vein problems and hemorrhoids but the oil is highly toxic, irritating, and can cause sun sensitivity.

Sage (*Salvia Officinalis*)

Although some religions consider sage a sacred herb, its uses go far beyond those in religion. Sage is a common shrub-like herb with rough, wrinkled leaves used as a spice. The oil is extracted by steam distillation and has been successfully used to treat menstrual problems, arthritis, bacterial infections, and as a sedative to treat insomnia. In high doses, the oil can lead to over stimulation of the brain and lead to epilepsy, described by the nonprofit Epilepsy Foundation of America as a brain disorder that produces seizures affecting a variety of mental and physical functions. When someone has two or more unprovoked seizures, he or she is considered epileptic.

Sassafras (*Sassafras albidum*)

Sassafras oil is steam distilled from the dried root barks of the deciduous tree that can grow to be as tall as 80 feet. It has slender branches, yellowish flowers, and a soft, spongy, orange-hued bark. Ancient herbalists used sassafras to treat arthritis, high blood pressure, kidney ailments, rheumatism, gout, and skin conditions. Sassafras oil unfortunately has about 80 to 90 percent safrole content, and as such, has been banned by the FDA because of its carcinogenic properties. Aside from the fact that using the oil can cause cancer, it is considered lethal even in small amounts.

Savory (*Satureja Hortensis, Satureja Montana*)

The two native English savory plants that bear the essential oil are *satureja hortensis*, also known as "summer savory," and *satureja montana*, also known as "mountain savory" or "winter savory." Both are fast growing plants that can be harvested within two months of sowing and used as savory culinary herbs for all groups of food — meats, poultry, fish, and vegetables. The only difference between the two savory plants is that summer savory is cultivated year-round unlike the winter savory that thrives in winter.

Savory oil, which is extracted by steam distillation, is highly irritating to the skin. Still, it has therapeutic properties, including being an antibacterial, antiseptic, antifungal, immune system stimulant, and a general tonic that can alleviate acute pain. Because of its high content of the naturally occurring compound phenol, the oil in very heavy dilutions is also used to speed up the formation of scar tissue and healing of burns and cuts.

Tansy (*Tanacetum Vulgare*)

The tansy perennial herb is native to Europe and is now often used as a hedgerow because of its agreeable height of no more than 3 feet as well as its alternating leaves. These leaves are called alternating because they grow on opposite sides of the stem. Its therapeutic uses benefit a variety of conditions including rheumatism and gout, but the oil distilled from tansy's leaves contain thujone, a poisonous compound that can cause convulsions, organ failure, vomiting, uterine bleeding, and respiratory arrest.

Wintergreen (*Gaultheria Procumbens*)

Wintergreen essential oil is steam distilled from the leaves of a small, creeping, evergreen shrub that is only 6 inches tall and can grow under trees and other shrubs. It is found in Canada and parts of the United States that have large sandy patches, barren plains, or mountainous tracts. The shrub bears droopy white flowers, stiff branches, and shiny oval leaves whose upper sides are a glossy bright green and undersides are dull green. Wintergreen oil is used in heavy dilutions to make ointments used for rheumatic conditions. The oil contains heavy amounts (98 percent) of methyl salicylate, a powerful toxin that is best avoided because it can cause blistering and swelling on areas of the skin to which it is applied, the face, tongue, throat, and even cause breathing difficulties.

Wormseed (*Chenopodium Ambrosioides*)

Once useful in expelling parasitic roundworms and hookworms from the body, wormseed essential oil is now no longer used because of its harmful effects on the liver, kidneys, and heart. The essential oil comes from the seeds of *chenopodium ambrosioides*, a perennial weed native to Mexico that now grows in New England, Missouri, and other parts of the United States, mostly in waste and manure areas.

Wormwood (*Artemisia Absinthum*)

All parts of *artemisia absinthum* herb, almost as bitter as rue, can be used for essential oil extraction. It was supposedly used to make absinthe, the favorite drink of famous 19th century artist Vincent van Gogh, and is said to have caused him to experience auditory and visual hallucinations, among other unpleasant side effects that may have caused him to cut off one of his earlobes. The oil contains thujone, a toxin that can also cause convulsions.

Yellow Sweetclover
(*Melilotus Officinalis*)

This essential oil comes from an herbaceous legume grown for forage. It has leaves growing on both sides of the stem and yellow flowers. The plant has a characteristic fresh grass aroma that intensifies when dried. It contains coumarin, which is used as an ingredient in perfume and in the past was used as a food additive. That latter use is not recommended, because it has been found to be toxic on the liver and kidneys.

Essential oils have a myriad of other uses that you may never think are related to aromatherapy. These include their use in the home, for everyday tasks like cleaning. These uses are explored next.

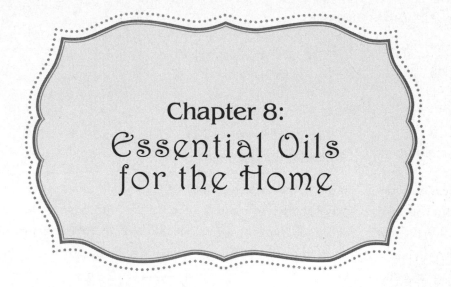

Chapter 8:
Essential Oils
for the Home

House cleaning is hardly an enjoyable activity for many of us. Parents do not like the chore any more than their children do, but you can make the experience more enjoyable if you clean your bedroom, studio, or home without coughing or eye irritation due to chemical-laden cleaners. Essential oils can make the job easier, because they are unlikely to make your cleaning experience hazardous. You can concoct safe and fragrant cleaning solutions using essential oils to clean every surface in your home and always remember to label them.

All-Purpose Cleaners

It is easy to make a safe, yet effective, all-purpose cleaner you can use on your floors, kitchen, bedroom, and bathroom. If you do not have any experience mixing cleaning chemicals or essential oils, your nose can assist you with this task.

Gather the following materials to make your cleaner:

- Your choice of essential oil
- Baking soda

- Distilled vinegar

- Purified water

- A spray bottle that ideally is not plastic

To make this cleaner:

- Add eight to ten drops of essential oil to 1 gallon purified water, 1 cup of distilled vinegar, and ½ ounce of baking soda.

Lemon is one of the safest, most effective cleaning and disinfecting essential oils but depending on personal preference and comfort, you can substitute it or blend it with tea tree, lavender, or another essential oil of choice. The acidic nature of lemon juice works to cut through any grime invading your home.

Disinfectants and Mold Treatments

You will not find essential oils singularly listed by the U.S. Environmental Agency (EPA) as effective disinfectants or mold treatments, but you will find products that contain essential oils, like factory-manufactured soap. Essential oils such as balsam of Peru, cinnamon, clove, lavender, lemon, lime, rosemary, tea tree, and thyme have strong antiseptic qualities and are good disinfectants against the EPA-identified pathogens. Use a mixture of just 1 teaspoon of any of these essential oils with 2 cups of purified water in a spray bottle to disinfect surfaces in your home, office, and even hospital room.

When it comes to mold treatment, you should first understand how prevalent and dangerous mold infections are. The results of a 2006 U.S. National Institutes of Health (NIH)-funded study published in the widely respected *Annals of Allergy, Asthma, and Immunology*, the official publication of the American College of Allergy, Asthma, & Immunology, found that more than half the homes in the United States have mold damage, most of it hidden from the homeowner's view. The study, conducted by a group of eight scientists and medical professionals from various institutions including the University of Cincinnati Department of Environmental Health and the National Risk Management Research Laboratory in North Carolina, sought to find answers for how water damage in homes result in mold and how often infants in these homes are affected with lower tract respiratory illnesses, such as bronchitis, as a result. The study also investigated why these infants' parents are atopic, meaning they develop hypersensitive reactions like dermatitis or asthma in parts of the body not in contact with the mold. The results of the study, titled "Mold Damage in Homes and Wheezing in Infants," were based on 640 home visits across the United States.

Microscopic mold spores can be found in general dust around the home but they only grow, multiply, and infect if the conditions are right. For example, spilled water on the carpet that is not dry in 48 hours allows the opportunistic mold fungi to settle in and start multiplying. Such affected carpeting would normally have to be replaced or be professionally cleaned but luckily, essential oils such as clove, eucalyptus, and tea tree that disinfect your home can also kill mold-causing fungi. To make a mixture to help combat mold, combine 2 teaspoons of essential oil and 2 cups of warm water to turn your home or office into a hostile environment for these fungi.

Glass Cleaners

You are probably happy with and even fond of your blue, store-bought glass cleaner. As difficult as it is to consider replacing your glass cleaner, think about its contents. Any person who has ever used commercially available window cleaners knows that it contains ammonia, an irritant that can cause some discomfort and damage to the eyes and other mucus membranes. Commercial glass cleaners also contain butyl cellusolve, a toxin that can depress the nervous system, while others contain glycol ethers, solvents that can cause anemia if used for a lengthy period spanning several years.

The sad thing about placing yourself and your family at such risk is that you really do not have to use these glass cleaners. Alternatively, we can easily create safer glass cleaners using natural products like essential oils.

For streak-free glass surfaces, combine the following ingredients:

• Three drops of peppermint essential oil

• Six drops of lemon essential oil

• ¾ cup of distilled vinegar

• ¼ cup of water

Some recipes call for ½ teaspoonful of Borax, a natural compound available from the grocery store that contains alkali and is good for cleaning; however, the recipe works just as well without Borax. You can also double or triple the measurements for a solution you can use multiple times.

Cream Cleaners

Cream cleaners are used to remove the dirt, grime, and makeup that we accumulate on our faces and bodies every day without subjecting ourselves to harsh chemicals. You can use simple essential oil cream cleanser recipes to make your own products.

To make a soothing cream cleanser, you will need:

• 1 tablespoon of heavy cream

• 1 drop of essential oil

Some of the best essential oils for this mixture include carrot seed oil or rose oil while avocado oil makes a functional base. You can also choose essential oils based on your skin type and texture and whether your skin can tolerate them.

Precautions

The skin on your face tends to be more sensitive than skin on other parts of your body. When using any essential oil on your face, make sure that it is properly diluted. Also make sure that you are not sensitized to the essential oil you are using to avoid adverse reactions. You should also ensure the oil is not phototoxic, which would require you to avoid exposure to sunlight for periods of more than two hours.

Cleaning Floors and Carpets

Grease on the kitchen floor can be tricky to clean; however, using essential oil mixtures can easily cut the grease, leaving your floors squeaky clean and smelling good. These mixtures can also be used for other floors, including your bathroom. Recommended essential oils for floor cleaners include eucalyptus, lemon, pine, and sweet orange with a measurement of ten drops of essential oil per gallon of water.

To make your hardwood floors sparkle, mix together:

- Ten drops of peppermint essential oil

- ¾ cup of vinegar

- ¾ cup of water

Carpets require frequent freshening, especially when there are pets or young children in a home that can respectively leave fleas and stains. To clean your carpet, mix ten drops of lavender essential oil for each gallon of water you use in your carpet cleaner. To deodorize and disinfect your carpet, mix together:

- Ten drops of tea tree essential oil

- Ten drops of lemon essential oil

- 3 tablespoonfuls of distilled vinegar

- 2 teaspoonfuls of Borax

- 16 ounces of baking soda

Stain Removers

Your favorite red wine on your favorite white blouse or shirt makes for a bad combination but thankfully not always a permanent one. If you happen to spill on yourself or on the carpet, immediately wash off and rinse the stain with club soda then soak the clothing in 4 tablespoons of Borax, 4 cups of cold water, and two drops of an essential oil such as lemon. It is a safe alternative to bleach, which often leaves behind an unpleasant smell and can quickly deteriorate clothing.

For carpet stain removal, lavender, lemon, or tea tree essential oils mixed with a few other ingredients can work well. A basic mixture should include:

- 2 tablespoons of Borax
- ½ cup of distilled vinegar
- 3 cups of hot water
- Three drops of an essential oil of your choice

Rub this mixture into the stain, let it dry, and vacuum it up. The process might need to be repeated if the stain is not removed to your satisfaction.

Home Deodorizers

Homes can sometimes develop the most unpleasant smells. Smells from the family dog, your children's play clothes, or even the odor from dinner two nights ago can overtake a home. A simple recipe for a home deodorizer requires only:

- A clean 16 ounce spray bottle full of water
- ½ cup of baking soda
- Ten to 12 drops of an essential oil of your choice

Some suggestions for essential oils to try include eucalyptus, pine, lavender, lemon, grapefruit, and rosemary.

Air freshening

You can easily and inexpensively make air fresheners using essential oils to refresh your whole home. Use them to spray your drapes and other areas while taking care to avoid wooden surfaces, because these sprays are more water-based and water can damage wood.

You can create concoctions of various air freshening scents using one simple recipe. These scents make up the seven groups of essential oils — citrus, earthy, floral, herbal, minty, spicy, and woody. To make an aromatic air freshener, add:

- 15 drops of an essential oil of your choice, either one from the groups or a blended mixture

- ½ teaspoon of vodka

Add the ingredients to a 16-ounce spray bottle with water in it. The vodka makes the concoction last longer, but water can be used for smaller quantities that can be used up on the same day.

Potpourri

If you are making your own potpourri, you can get all the raw materials you need from your backyard or your local florist. Strike a rapport with florists to allow you to scoop up their damaged flowers, which you can then mix with the other plant materials you have collected. All these then have to be dried, either in the sun for several days, or using a dehydrator. You can then blend four or more essential oils for a desired aroma.

Add your blend of essential oils to a dark-colored glass bottle and mix with the dried up plant material. Each time the aroma in the bottle dissipates, add a few more drops of your essential oil blend to freshen up the mixture. Try making blends of essential oils or absolutes considered to be "fixatives," because they prevent volatile oils and their aromas from evaporating quickly. Fixatives are heavily viscous oils such as balsam of Peru, benzoin, cedarwood, frankincense, myrrh patchouli, sandalwood, and vanilla oleoresin.

To scent your potpourri, put your assortment of plant material in a glass bowl and add ten drops of your essential oil blend. Feel free to adjust the amount of drops that go into the potpourri assortment depending on how much you have and the strength you want for your potpourri. Each time the scent in your potpourri weakens, just add more drops of your essential oil to freshen the aroma. This simple concoction makes a wonderful air freshener for your home or office.

CASE STUDY: ANYA WOLFENDEN

Director of Communications
The Heritage Store: Natural Foods,
Cafe, Bookstore, and Holistic Center
Virginia Beach, Va.
757-428-0500
www.heritagestore.com
www.caycecures.com

A veteran public speaker, Anya Wolfenden has designed seminars for more than 25 years and has spoken on radio, television, and to groups as varied as DC Arts and Cultural Alliance to the U.S. Navy, International Herb Association, and Eastern Virginia Medical School about creative well-being, aromatherapy, and nutritional health. She is also a food and wellness columnist, an author, and she teaches intricate, hands-on classes on aromatherapy.

Wolfenden was introduced to aromatherapy and essential oils more than 20 years ago while working as a massage therapist. She then studied on her own to further her knowledge. "I had a natural orientation and when I started working with essential oils, I began to incorporate them in my life by making anything from bug repellent to house cleaners and pet shampoos."

The mother of two daughters loves the many practical ways to use essential oils to help alleviate minor ailments like joint pain, headaches, and insomnia. With access to a lab at The Heritage Store, Wolfenden is part of the team that formulates wonderful products, like a poultice called Alka-Thyme that contains eucalyptus oil, among other ingredients, and is good for soothing the lymph nodes, sinus infections, and chest congestions.

Wolfenden says that though these treatments are not FDA approved, she believes they work.

"Essential oils are the lifeblood of the plants and they have pharmacological, physiological, and physical aspects that we should all respect."

Essential Oils for Your Laundry

Instead of rushing out to buy new detergent to keep your clothes and linens smelling fresh and clean, all you have to do is add your favorite essential oils to your laundry. Begin by loading your clothes in your washing machine. Mix unscented natural laundry soap with three to five drops of an essential oil such as lavender and add the mixture to the washing machine, letting the load wash normally. The scent of the essential oils you use are likely to remain on your clothes if you use low heat or line dry your now perfect-smelling clothes.

Fabric softeners

Feel free to blend essential oils for your homemade fabric softener. To get started, gather the following ingredients:

- 1 cup baking soda
- 6 cups distilled white vinegar
- 6 cups water
- 15 drops essential oils

Adjust the quantity of the essential oil depending on whether you are using more than one. You can then use the mixture like you would use any store bought fabric softener.

Cleaning Your Dishes

Essential oils such as bergamot, orange, pine, spruce, and tangerine can enhance the fragrance of your liquid dishwashing soap and disinfect them. One or two drops is all you need for a load of dishes and they rinse easily and completely, leaving no residue for you to taste next time you use your dishes or silverware. Exercise caution, because frequently using essential oils in your dishwasher is not recommended because they can degrade the plastic parts inside the machine.

Furniture Cleaning

The same mixture you used to deodorize your home can also deodorize your furniture. The mixture can also kill dust mites that tend to be everywhere humans are — in sofas and mattresses for instance. They are microscopic eight-legged critters that feed off the dead skin we shed every day and can cause allergies.

You can also easily make your own furniture polish to substitute for the phenol-laced polish found in stores. Store bought polish contains nitrobenzene, a toxic chemical absorbed through the skin that can cause breathing problems, birth defects, liver problems, and may be a carcinogen. To make your safe furniture polish, mix the following ingredients into a 16-ounce spray bottle filled with purified water:

- 2 teaspoons extra virgin olive oil
- ¼ cup of distilled vinegar
- 12 to 15 drops of an essential oil like lemon

Lemon oil is the safest and most versatile oil to use on all kinds of surfaces. It can help keep your wood surfaces from looking dry and faded. You may want to avoid cinnamon oil on wooden surfaces, because it has a tendency to leave stains.

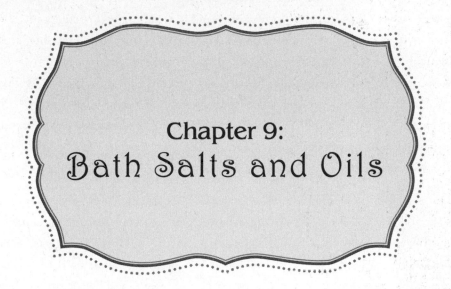

Chapter 9:
Bath Salts and Oils

Taking a bath is probably one of the simplest activities many of us can enjoy without spending much money. Adding bath oils and bath salts to your bathing experience can only enhance your enjoyment and using essential oils has the added bonus of being therapeutic.

Bath Salts

Citrus and floral bath salts are more popular perhaps because of their invigorating aromas and because they are as easy to make as they are to enjoy. However, try indulging in other essential oil categories when creating your bath salts. All you need to create therapeutic, invigorating, aromatic, and natural bath salts begins with the simple recipe of adding 20 to 30 drops of one or more essential oils to 16 ounces of natural bath salt. Bath salts are available from local and online retailers like SaltWorks (**www.saltworks.us**), a Seattle-based salt company that carries wonderfully natural salts in many different varieties. In fact, the company proudly states on its website that it offers more than 110 varieties of gourmet salts from around the world and maintains an inventory of more than 4 million pounds.

Good bath salts can be either fine or coarse and have naturally occurring minerals, such as magnesium and potassium, that do good things for your body including reducing high blood pressure and aiding in metabolism. Because they increase water salinity, they also decrease the bacteria count on your skin, thereby helping your body maintain a stronger, more efficient immune system. Additionally, bath water enriched with soluble bath salts and essential oils works as a natural scrub against your skin, exfoliating dead and damaged skin while offering important therapeutic effects, not just for the body, but for the mind, too.

Do not limit your creativity when creating homemade bath salts. Consider adding homemade potpourri or fresh flower petals to your bathtub to enhance the inevitably enjoyable experience of using refreshing and invigorating bath salts. Always try to add your essential oil-laden concoctions to your bath water just before you get into the tub. This allows you to reap the full benefits of their properties rather than watch or smell them evaporate into thin air. Remember that essential oils are volatile and evaporate quickly.

Difference Between Bombs and Salts

Unlike bath salts that resemble kitchen salt both in appearance and no fuss solubility, bath bombs are meant to be fizzy when they react to your bath water. One of their most important qualities is their effervescence, which is very similar to popular antacids such as Alka-Seltzer but on a grander scale.

Bath bombs

To create a basic bath bomb for someone with oily or blemished skin, gather some baking soda, citric acid, fragrant essential oil, round molds, and a spray bottle of witch hazel, an essential oil with powerful astringent properties that make it useful in controlling oiliness and skin blemishes. For strictly aesthetic purposes, you can also add a coloring additive like mica powder, which is available in several different shades. You can use this recipe for all types of skin, substituting only the essential oil. For instance, you can use ylang-ylang and rose geranium to make a moisturizing bath bomb that will leave your skin soft and nourished.

How to make a bath bomb

For your homemade bomb, carefully combine the following ingredients:

INGREDIENTS

2 cups baking soda

1 cup citric acid found in lemon juice

20 to 25 drops of an essential oil of your choice

Coloring (as much or as little as you prefer)

DIRECTIONS

1. Combine these ingredients in a clean, preferably glass container.

2. Using a mold — one made out of stainless steel or plastic— is optional but recommended for an even, smooth blend.

3. Add the essential oil drop by drop, all the while stirring the mixture. If the mixture gets to be too hard, spray it with the witch hazel to moisten it up. Remember to keep mixing your ingredients. You can even use your hands to aid the mixture.

4. Mix the combination until it is well blended with the right consistency — not too moist — at which point you will begin to place the mixture into the molds, paying attention so as not to waste any.

5. Once the mixture is tightly packed in the molds, allow them to air dry for about four hours. The results are round, hard, bath bombs that are ready to be dropped into your tub and indulge your need for a soothing and relaxing bath.

Bath Oils

You can give the Avon lady a run for her money by canceling your next appointment and creating your own therapeutic and skin-enhancing bath oils. A basic recipe calls for 15 to 20 drops of an essential oil or a blend of essential oils in a 2 ounce base carrier.

To mix the bath oils, add carrier oil into a dark-colored glass bottle and then add essential oils drop by drop. Tightly close the bottle and store it away from sunlight and artificial light whenever it is not in use. To use your bath oils, add 1 or 2 teaspoons of bath oil per bath. Make sure you know how your skin tolerates each essential oil used to make your bath oils and be even more careful if your skin is sensitive or if you allow children to use the mixture.

Special herbal baths

Herbs like clary sage, rosemary, thyme, and yarrow can be dried whole and placed in a clean cloth with a string tying up the ends, or inside an old sock, to use in the bath tub. A basic recipe calls for just 3 cups of herbs recommended for use in a very hot bath. You should allow this herb mixture to steep for 30 minutes to an hour. Alternatively, the bag of herbs can be submerged in a boiling pot of water and left to steep for 30 minutes before adding the herb-infused water to an already drawn bath. The latter method has some drawbacks because it can let volatile essential oils contained in the dried plants to escape, thus minimizing the therapeutic benefits of the brew.

Chapter 10:
Making Soap

Soap is probably one of the most frequently used body care tools and the least understood in terms of its ingredients. This chapter will help you understand the various aspects of soap, how its made, and how to make it fun.

What is Soap?

Understanding what soap is does not require a trip to the chemistry lab. Although there is a science to what soap is that involves knowledge of compounds, the compounds' water solubility, and the role heat and oxygen play, all you need to know is that soap is a combination of water, **alkali** (lye made from wood ash), and acid (vegetable oils or animal fats). These ingredients combine to create a chemical reaction called **saponification**, which is the splitting of the oils or fats into their two natural parts — fatty acids and glycerin. The process neutralizes the alkali and the end result is soap, to which you can add essential oils, color, and additives such as oatmeal.

Introduction to Soap Making

Soap is one of the universal things used around the world. Today, soap is commercially available very inexpensively and thus very little focus is placed on soap making as a necessity. But did you know that making your own soaps could be a very invigorating, creative, and therapeutic process? To fully understand this process, let us first understand how it began.

History of Soap Making

It is impossible to deny the influence soap has had on human civilization. What is unclear is when soap actually became such an important part of everyday human lives. Some theories conclude that prehistoric humans were the original makers and users of soap but some conclude that the Gauls living in what is now Belgium and France are responsible for soap, especially goats' milk soap recipes. Other accounts credit ancient Greeks with using wood ashes (primitive lye) to clean their pots and cherished statues of Greek gods. Roman legend has the origin of soap as accidental. When they sacrificed animals on Mount Sapo, animal fats and wood ashes, guided by rain water, trickled down Mount Sapo to the Tiber River where women washing clothes found the mixture to be useful in cleaning their garments. In Africa, wood ashes gathered after cooking in open fires, were mixed with water and used to clean pots and other items before it was discovered that adding animal fats to the mixture was even better. Wood ashes, when mixed with fats or oils, produces a chemical reaction called saponification. This process results in the soaps used every day.

After these discoveries came soap factories. The first one is said to have been in Marseilles, France, where olive oil was used to make what is known as castile soap, which was all the rage before the introduction of palm and cocoa oils. Nicholas Le Blanc, a French chemist and physician, is credited with revolutionizing soap making by developing the Le Blanc process, an industrial way to produce soda ash, also known as sodium carbonate. He developed the process in 1791 in response to a French Academy of Sciences offer for prize money to the individual(s) who could come up with a way to produce alkali from sea salt. James Muspratt, a British chemical manufacturer, introduced the Le Blanc process to England during the 1810s, and in 1811 Michel-Eugene Chevreul, a French chemist, identified the exact measurements of fat necessary to make soap, helping the industry and art develop into an exact science.

Today, commercial soap making features advanced technologies. These include machines that produce large amounts of soap by allowing soap manufacturers to add ingredients on one end of the machine, allowing the chemical reactions needed to produce soap to take place at one end of the machine, and producing the finished product on the other end of the machine. Soap making at home, on the other hand, follows the unchanged recipe that the Romans might have accidentally discovered: water, fat, and an alkali to make soap.

Making Your Own Soap

Whether you are looking for a natural alternative to the everyday soaps available on grocery store shelves, you are a chemistry lover looking for a new experience, or you are just someone simply looking to try natural products, soap making can be a satisfying activity. To get started, you should first understand and gather the kind of equipment necessary.

Equipment

There are several tools of the trade that make the process of soap making much easier and safer. You should consider buying the following items for making your own soaps:

- An accurate scale or other measuring equipment is integral, because wrong measurements can produce undesirable consistencies

- A thermometer

- Wooden molds

- Soap cutters

- Freezer paper to line your molds

- Pots and pans to mix your ingredients

- Ladles

- Spatulas

- A source of heat to melt your animal fats

- Safety gear such as aprons, gloves, and goggles

All this equipment can be found at a local hardware store, grocery store, or online store.

For safety

Any time you are using alkali, which is a caustic chemical compound that can burn the skin and corrode some surfaces, you want to make sure that you have taken necessary precautions to protect yourself and those around you. For soap making, the alkali in the lye, a necessary ingredient, mandates the use of goggles to protect your eyes, gloves to protect your hands and arms, an apron to protect your clothes, vinegar to neutralize lye just in case you spill it on a patch of skin, and a well ventilated area to allow you to breath less caustic fumes.

Pots and pans

Pots and pans are necessary when you are making soap at home, because the soap making process involves heating some ingredients. Large 12-quart stainless steel pots and pans are preferable, because they are less likely to add contaminants to your mixtures and are more durable against the corrosive effects of lye. Once you designate pots and pans for soap making, you should not use them for cooking to eliminate the chances of getting lye in your food.

Scales and measuring equipment

If you have a recipe that calls for 5.6 ounces of lye and you inadvertently use 6.5 ounces of lye, the finished product may have too much alkali and thus be overly harsh. Similarly, a recipe that calls for 4 ounces of coconut oil that ends up having

8 ounces or just 2 ounces can lead to either an over fattened or hard product that does not clean as well or is overly drying to your skin.

An accurate measuring device is the best investment you can make to benefit your soap making activities. A scale that measures in 1 ounce increments and has a minimum capacity of at least 10 pounds will allow you to make soap in adequate batches. Pyrex bowls that are heat resistant and have quart measurements can also come in handy for your liquid measurements. For ingredients you will need in smaller quantities, such as essential oils, a stainless steel teaspoon will serve as a functional measuring device.

Utensils

These include the ladles and spoons you will use to mix you ingredients, spatulas to help you scoop out every bit of your mixture from the pot to the mold, and soap cutters to cut the finished product into manageable sizes. Your wooden ladles and spoons should come in a variety of sizes to be used as necessary.

Molds

Molds allow your finished product to take shape. They allow you to be creative and decorative with your shapes. Wooden molds lined with freezer paper work best, because they are more resistant to lye corrosion and can therefore last longer, but you can use plastic molds if you spray them with cooking spray.

Miscellaneous

Stainless steel thermometers are useful to ensure that your mixture is maintaining the temperature your recipe calls for. However, thermometers are not necessary to cold process soaps, which do not contain animal fat that may need to be melted. You can use towels or blankets to insulate your mixture while it cures in the mold for anywhere from a few hours to few weeks. Once you gather these essential equipment pieces, you can then set off on the next phase of your soap making adventure by first beginning to gather the necessary ingredients.

Ingredients

Each ingredient that goes into making soap should complement what your plan to use the soap for. For example, if the soap will be used for cleaning the face, you probably want a gentler soap than the one you would want to use to clean floors, so you will want to use less lye in your face soap. Soap that will be used to clean an auto mechanic's oil-covered body after a full day of work will probably have more sodium hydroxide than soap to be used by a beauty queen who just scored a crown. These ingredients all work in concert to create what could be the best soap you ever use.

For a successful experience, use a basic soap recipe that you can then expand on as you become more knowledgeable. All you need is animal fat (tallow) or vegetable oil, lye, and cold water.

Lye

Lye, also called an alkali base, is a caustic substance that causes the chemical reactions necessary to make soap. Lye is available commercially, but the adventurous can make lye right in their kitchens. The process is simple but it can be daunting for a novice, because getting the right consistency of strength for your lye and consequently for your soap may be difficult. All you need to make lye is water and wood ash, preferably from hardwood trees like ash, beech, birch, buckeye, cherry, elm, or maple. Hardwoods are less resinous than softwoods and are easier to mix with fat and vegetable oils for good quality soap.

Water

Soap making works best with soft water that is devoid of excess impurities and minerals. You should invest in a good water purification system to make sure you remove the impurities. The best way to tell if your water is soft enough is to check whether your newly minted soap does not rinse off easily when you use it.

Purified water

Do you ever wonder about the cleanliness of the water that comes out of your faucets? Each city, town, or county has a water purification system that at some point includes the wastewater treatment facility. You may naturally worry that not every harmful organism is killed during the treatment process, but purifying the water that comes out of your faucet can help calm your worries.

Tap water

Tap water tends to be hard water because of excessive minerals like calcium and magnesium, which tap water picks up during the purification process. Unless it is de-mineralized before you use it, tap water can produce cloudy soap that does not lather well. The process of demineralization removes these minerals from the water by a process called reverse osmosis that involves passing the hard water through a special membrane available at home improvement stores. This membrane captures these minerals but allows demineralized water to pass through.

Seawater

Seawater not only has salt but is said to be nutrient rich with compounds such as potassium that help in overall body wellness. Seawater is thus unmatched in the benefits it can offer your skin when used in soap making. When you want soap with antibacterial, antifungal, and anti-inflammatory properties, seawater is at the top of the list of recommendations. You can harness seawater directly from the sea or buy it from vitamin stores.

Well water

Well water tends to be soft but it can also contain natural minerals found deep under the surface. To see if you can use your well water to make soap, make a small batch; then try to make the soap foam. If it foams easily, the well water is fine to use as it is. If it does not foam up easily, you can make it usable by adding baking soda a tablespoon or two at a time to your water and soap mixture. Stir the mixture until the baking soda disappears and keep adding baking soda until the soap foams easily. Although this process may seem like a lengthy one, consider that it only needs to be done once.

Rainwater

This is soft water because it does not contain minerals that can be metallic or acidic chemicals. You can easily collect rainwater by catching it using a rain barrel or large buckets. You do not have to purify or distill rain water for soap making, but sometimes you might have to strain it to make sure unwanted leaves or tiny branches do not make it into your soap mixture.

Scented water

This can be scented with essential oils, synthetic fragrance, flower petals, or herbs. Once you have made sure the water is soft by making sure it lathers well, add your scent. When using essential oils, add ten drops to each cup of water, avoiding top note essential oils that evaporate quickly and lose their fragrance. You can use this mixture immediately to make your soap.

When using flower petals, ½ cup of flower petals like those from roses is sufficient in 2 cups of water. When using herbs, 1 cup of herbs like sage in 1 quart of water will do. You can adjust these quantities depending on how strong or weak you want your scent solution to be. Let the mixtures steep for up to seven days, then strain them before use.

Milk

Milk can replace water in your soap mixture and produce wonderfully creamy soaps. Many varieties exist but the most popular milk used for soap making is goat's milk for its creamy and moisturizing properties and coconut milk for its creamy bubbles. You can also use cow's milk, buttermilk, or coconut milk.

Extra vigilance is needed when using milk instead of water. The sugars found in milk react differently to lye than water. As the lye heats up, it can scorch the sugars, turning the milk brown. This does not affect the final product negatively other than giving your soap a light brown coloring, but if you do not like the change in color you can minimize this reaction by making sure your mixture does not heat up beyond 100 degrees Fahrenheit.

Infusions

Infusions are botanical matter like herbs and flowers steeped in hot water for about 30 minutes, or in cold water or oil for up to seven days, to extract their beneficial properties for use in soap making. Chamomile, lavender, and peppermint are popular herbs used in infusions. You can even use brewed tea, like chamomile, for your lye solution instead of plain water.

Fats and oils

Fats from most animals can be used in soap making but the most popular, perhaps because of their familiarity, are fats from cattle and lard from pigs. Those who are very adventurous can prepare their own fats by separating the meat from the fat, chopping up the fat, melting it over low heat, and "washing" it by scraping off any dirt that remains after the melted fat has cooled. Oils are liquid at room temperature and can be either from animals, like those from fish, or plant and vegetable based. The latter are preferred by those who have qualms about using animal products.

Note: Each pound of fat produces about one 1 cup of grease, which has to be strained through a cheesecloth.

Animal Versus Vegetable Base

As the push toward vegetarianism and veganism has gained popularity and the use of animal byproducts has become somewhat unpopular, soap making has evolved from using just animal fats to using oils extracted from vegetables, grains, and nuts. Soaps made with vegetable oils are said to be chemically superior to soaps made with animal fats, because the skin readily absorbs vegetable oils while animal fats can clog pores and result in skin conditions such as acne.

The types of fats and oils you use also determine how quickly your soap begins to form. Animal fats allow your soap mixture to saponify quickly, or reach trace faster. The term **"reaching trace"** refers to the moment that your soap mixture turns into a pudding- or gravy-like state. With animal fats, your mixture can begin to saponify in 30 minutes to an hour, whereas lighter oils like vegetable oils can take several hours to several days.

Animal fats can also achieve false trace if the mixture is left at room temperature, allowing the fats to solidify. To avoid this, these fats need to be at temperatures that allow them to remain in liquid form.

Oils to Use When Making Soaps

There are a wide variety of oils and fats that you can use in your soap making adventures to produce superior soaps. Keep in mind that soaps can retain some of the scents, hues, nutrients, and therapeutic properties of the essential oils used.

Almond (sweet) oil

This soap-making oil is often used for super fattened soaps, which are soaps meant to be very moisturizing. Adding extra oil to a soap mixture after it has traced allows the oil to bypass the saponification process and maintain most or all of its oily benefits and properties. You can use almond oil at 10 to 15 percent in combination with coconut oil or palm oil.

CHARACTERISTICS AND BENEFITS

Super fattened sweet almond soap is mild, super soft, and creamy with very stable lather. It does not produce a quick trace but once it sets, it is a great moisturizer. Almond oil is often used in lip balms, which leave lips soft and luscious.

Avocado oil

Avocado oil is popular in soap making because it contains a high percentage of unsaponifiable molecules, many of which are nutrients that do not combine with the lye and therefore remain intact in the final product. Avocado oil does not speed up trace and can be used in combination with shea butter, castor, and coconut oils, using just 5 to 10 percent of avocado oil in your oils mixture. For instance, if your recipe calls for 30 ounces of fats and oils, you should not use more than 3 ounces of avocado oil. You should then use other oils to satisfy the remaining 27 ounces.

CHARACTERISTICS AND BENEFITS

Avocado oil soap is soft with mild cleansing properties. It creates a stable, creamy lather but is not reliable for bubbles. Use avocado oil in combination with other oils such as coconut or palm oil to avoid a soap that is too soft and dissolves prematurely. Soap made out of avocado oil is good for dry skin, helping it retain moisture.

Calendula oil

Soap recipes that call for the use of calendula oil often suggest that you infuse olive oil with ground calendula petals, but for a beginner, you will probably find it easier to just use calendula oil obtained from a natural or health food store. You only need 10 percent of calendula oil in combination with coconut oil, palm oil, or olive oil. The best way to obtain the benefits of calendula oil is to add it at trace to prevent the lye mixture from changing the oil's nutrients.

CHARACTERISTICS AND BENEFITS

Calendula oil soap is a soft soap with creamy, lotion-like lather and mild cleaning capabilities. It has anti-inflammatory benefits that are especially good for those with damaged, dry, or scaly skin. It is recommended for use by those with sensitive skin, especially babies.

Canola oil

Canola oil soap is slow to trace because it is less of a saturated fat. To speed up trace, use it at 50 percent in combination with palm oil, coconut oil, or sunflower oil. Canola oil is an excellent replacement to olive oil, which tends to be more expensive

CHARACTERISTICS AND BENEFITS

Apart from its affordability, canola oil soap is a good moisturizer and conditioner. If canola oil is used alone, the resulting soap is very soft, but this can be easily remedied by adding oil such as coconut oil that produces hard soap.

Castor oil

This oil is very appealing to use in soap making because it speeds up trace, decreasing the amount of time it takes for your ingredients to turn into soap, and because it creates a bubble-rich soap. Castor oil may be used in combination with coconut, grapeseed, olive, and palm oils.

CHARACTERISTICS AND BENEFITS

Castor oil produces a soft, creamy, and mild soap. Additionally, if you like soap with bubbly lather, use castor oil as an ingredient. Castor oil is effective in moisturizing your skin. Considering that it is used in lip balms and lipstick, it can easily make soap glide on skin while attracting and retaining moisture.

Cocoa butter oil

Unrefined cocoa butter oil produces a nice chocolate-like scent in your soap, while refined cocoa butter soap is unscented. Cocoa butter oil is a saturated fat that can make up to 15 percent of your total base oils in combination with apricot kernel oil, olive, or palm oil. It traces quickly and can also be used in equal amounts in combination with shea butter for a luxuriously soft soap.

CHARACTERISTICS AND BENEFITS

Cocoa butter oil works best when used as a super fattening oil. The soap has rich lather, is a firm soap, yet is very soft and moisturizing to the skin. Cocoa butter soap can last up to two years, because the antioxidants found in it prevent rancidity.

Coconut oil

Coconut oil is a saturated fat that can be used in soap making in combination with olive and palm oils. Although coconut oil makes soaps lather well, it can be drying to soap when it makes up more than 30 percent of the base oils used in your soap. It speeds up trace in your soap-making mixture.

CHARACTERISTICS AND BENEFITS

Coconut oil soap is hard and lathers exceedingly well, even when used in hard water. It suds up even when used in saltwater, and it is a strong cleanser so it works well to cut through tough grease and grime. Different types of coconut oil exist in soap making, including 76-degree coconut oil, 92-degree coconut oil, fractionated coconut oil, and virgin coconut oil.

- **76-degree coconut oil:** This oil melts at 76 degrees and is responsible for producing hard, bar soap and great lather.

- **92-degree coconut oil:** It melts at 92 degrees and is more hydrogenated and cheaper than the previous oil. Some soap makers prefer it because it is easier to scoop and requires minimal exertion. This kind of oil produces bar soap that is harder than the one produced using the 76-degree oil although it does not lather as well.

- **Fractionated coconut oil:** This oil is chemically altered by the removal of its medium chain of triglycerides. These fats are the chemical forms of fat that can then be used in making other products, including make up. Fractionated oil is so named because it only contains a fraction of the original fat found in coconut oil. It is considered saturated fat because its carbon atoms are fully saturated with hydrogen atoms, making it a solid at room temperature. One of its advantages in soap making is that it has a longer shelf life and can withstand greater heat.

- **Virgin coconut oil:** This comes from freshly grated coconut and is more costly, even though it has not been found to produce soap that is superior to those produced by the other types of coconut oil. Its use is better suited to use when making food than making soap but when so used, it makes hard, well lathering soap.

Cottonseed

Soap makers suggest using organic cottonseed oil, because it comes from seeds grown without the use of pesticides. Non-organic cotton is heavily sprayed, because it is not classified as an edible crop and also because insects frequently attack the crop. Pesticide residue is said to sometimes be present in cottonseed oil and this residue can be a carcinogen. It does not produce a quick trace and you can use it in combination with soybean oil at about 25 percent.

CHARACTERISTICS AND BENEFITS

Soap produced using cottonseed oil is soft and mild with a creamy lather but no bubbly lather. Because cottonseed oil does not have a long shelf life, its use in soap should be taken into consideration. The soap does have good moisturizing properties.

Hazelnut oil

Hazelnut oil produces soap that has several benefits and a short shelf life of six months at maximum. Adding rosemary oil to the hazelnut oil can help prolong the shelf life by a few more months. It does not trace quickly on its own but can be used in combination with other quick tracing oils and fats like tallow. Use no more than 5 percent of this oil in your total oils batch if you want to speed up trace.

CHARACTERISTICS AND BENEFITS

Hazelnut soap is hard with a stable lather and good cleansing abilities. It is an excellent moisturizer with astringent properties that help shrink pores, leaving skin tight and smooth.

Hemp seed oil

Like hazelnut oil, hemp seed oil has a short shelf life that can be extended by adding oils with longer shelf lives. Use hemp seed oil in combination with palm, castor oil, and shea butter at 15 percent of your total oils batch.

CHARACTERISTICS AND BENEFITS

Hemp seed soap is semi-hard with good, stable lathering capabilities. The oil contains anti-aging and anti-inflammatory properties that can also be found in the soap. With frequent use, it can help repair irritated skin while keeping wrinkles at bay. It is also a good moisturizer.

Jojoba oil

Jojoba oil in your soap making ingredients makes trace happen quickly. If that presents a problem and you would like to slow the process down a bit, add the jojoba oil at trace instead of at the beginning of the soap making process. It is best if you only add 10 percent of this oil in your soap solution, because more than that will produce soap that is too soft and has poor lathering capabilities. Use it in combination with shea butter and olive oil.

CHARACTERISTICS AND BENEFITS

Jojoba oil is a soft soap that produces oil laden with many positive benefits that include extra fighting powers against extra dry skin and wrinkles. The soap made from unrefined jojoba oil has a red hue while the one made from refined jojoba oil is white. Both soaps are mild with creamy, stable lather and few bubbles.

Kukui nut oil

This popular Hawaiian oil can work well if used to superfat your soap, because its nutrients will not undergo a chemical reaction that could diminish their therapeutic properties. **Superfatting** means adding extra oil at trace so that the resulting soap is very moisturizing. Kukui nut oil does not produce fast trace and it can be used at 5 to 10 percent in combination with shea butter and coconut oil.

CHARACTERISTICS AND BENEFITS

Kukui nut oil soap is mild and soft with excellent conditioning and creamy, stable lather. It can alleviate dry and chapped skin, acne, eczema, and soothe sunburns. Kukui nut oil is also one of the more expensive base oils.

Lard

Lard is pork fat that is available widely from grocers and butchers. Soaps made using the cold process method can be made solely with 100 percent lard. Soaps made using the hot process, also discussed later, require just 30 to 40 percent lard in combination with vegetable oils such as coconut and palm. Lard produces a quick trace.

CHARACTERISTICS AND BENEFITS

Lard soap is a mild cleanser, hard, and very white. It has a creamy, stable lather, and a very small quantity of bubbles. Contrary to common belief that soap made with lard can clog the pores, you will find that it is very good for moisturizing the skin.

Olive oil

Unlike in cooking where extra virgin olive oil is recommended, in soap making, lower grades of olive oil are recommended, because olive oil has a quicker trace and can help cut down on the time needed to make your soap. You can use olive oil in a recipe without combining it with any other oils. This is unlike other recipes, which often call for several oils because each oil offers different benefits and properties to the soap. For instance, when you want a soap that lathers well and is soft, you would use coconut oil for lather together with olive oil.

CHARACTERISTICS AND BENEFITS

Soap made from olive oil is creamy and lathers well but is not bubbly. It is mild, soft, and is a good moisturizer that does not clog pores but leaves your skin supple and younger looking.

Palm kernel oil

Although it has some similarities to palm oil, palm kernel oil produces soap with properties that more closely resembles coconut oil. It is available as a partially hydrogenated fat and as a liquid. Do not use this oil as more than 20 to 30 percent of your total base oils, because it can be drying to the skin in larger percentages. It produces a quick trace and can be used in combination with coconut oil but be careful to adjust your lye amounts; this oil requires less than the amount of lye required by coconut oil.

CHARACTERISTICS AND BENEFITS

Palm kernel oil makes a hard soap that lathers and cleanses well while producing plenty of bubbles. Palm kernel oil can help firm up a soap recipe that is too soft while giving the soap a smooth texture.

Palm oil

Palm oil is also known as vegetable tallow because it produces soap that is similar to soap produced by beef tallow (also known as beef fat), including its hardness and creamy lather. The oil is saturated and has to be melted and stirred or shaken because it tends to separate in its solid form. Palm oil is good for quick trace. Use 20 to 30 percent palm oil in combination with coconut, olive, or safflower oil.

CHARACTERISTICS AND BENEFITS

Palm oil soap is mild, hard, produces a stable, creamy lather, and produces some bubbles. When used frequently, soap made with palm oil is healing to dry and sun-damaged skin.

Peanut oil

Peanut oil is available in both refined and unrefined varieties. The refined variety is stripped of the proteins that cause peanut allergies and is said to be safe for those with allergies to use. For safety purposes, however, it is better to consult with a physician before using any kind of peanut oil in your soap. Use about 20 percent of peanut oil for your total base oil amounts.

CHARACTERISTICS AND BENEFITS

Peanut oil is highly unsaturated with a short shelf life. Once the peanut oil in the soap goes rancid, your beautiful soap is likely to develop orange spots and an off smell. It produces a soft and mild soap with stable lather and good conditioning qualities, but it does not produce trace quickly.

Safflower oil

Safflower oil is cold pressed from the seeds of the safflower plant, which is a close relative of the sunflower plant. The oil is odorless and colorless so when used in soap making, the byproduct bears the same characteristics. Safflower oil can take days to trace, so its use is best if capped at 10 percent in combination with oils like olive and hemp seed.

CHARACTERISTICS AND BENEFITS

Safflower oil has high amounts of linoleic acid, which contributes to the regulation of body functions such as blood pressure, blood clotting, and immunity to infections. When used in soap making, safflower oils can impart these benefits to the user in addition to moisturizing the skin. Safflower oil has a shelf life of about three months but can be used in combination with oils like olive oil that have longer shelf lives. It produces a firm bar with great conditioning capabilities and stable lather.

Sesame oil

Sesame oil is very heavy but can be blended with lighter oils like grapeseed and almond if you prefer using a lighter oil mixture. It can also be used in combination with palm and sunflower oils at 10 percent of the total base oils.

CHARACTERISTICS AND BENEFITS

Sesame oil soap is soft, has stable lather, and is valuable for moisturizing and conditioning. Sesame oil has a strong, nutty aroma that can sometimes overpower the scent of your other ingredients so feel free to experiment with a small batch to make sure you like the scent in your soap. Alternately, blend sesame oil with other base oils to reduce the aroma.

Soybean oil

Soap made from soybean oil has similar characteristics to lard and tallow and offers an alternative for people, like vegans, who do not use animal by-products. You can use it in combination with coconut and olive oils.

CHARACTERISTICS AND BENEFITS

Soybean soap is soft and mild with creamy, stable but not bubbly lather. Soybean oil comes both as a liquid and as a solid because of hydrogenation, which rearranges the chemical structure of oils to turn them into solids. Neither the liquid nor the solid is responsible for producing quick trace. The liquid (non-hydrogenated) produces soap that has better conditioning properties but less lather than the solid form.

Sunflower oil

Sunflower oil traces slowly but can be used at 10 to 15 percent with avocado oil, canola oil, jojoba oil, olive oil, and sweet almond oil to speed up trace. This type of oil is often used to produce bars for the face, body, and the kitchen.

CHARACTERISTICS AND BENEFITS

Sunflower oil is rich in vitamin E and lecithin, which makes the soap an excellent cell regenerator and ideal for fighting off wrinkles and scarring. The soap is soft with creamy lather and good conditioning abilities.

Tallow

This is fat from beef, which like lard is more useful to the skin than it is damaging. Tallow soap cleans better when made in combination with palm oil. This is good for producing quick trace.

CHARACTERISTICS AND BENEFITS

Tallow soap is hard with mild cleaning properties and creamy, stable lather. You can use it to produce soap for use on your body or to wash your clothes with.

Wheat germ oil

Wheat germ oil can be used in combination with base oils like coconut and palm kernel at just 10 percent of your total oils batch. Its high vitamin E content makes it more resistant to light and heat and a good natural preservative when used in cosmetic products like soap.

CHARACTERISTICS BENEFITS

Wheat germ oil, a natural source of many beneficial properties as discussed in Chapter 3, is good for treatment of eczema and psoriasis as well as for smoothing cracked, dehydrated, and wrinkled skin. Wheat germ oil soap is hardy with stable, full lather and good conditioning capabilities.

Super Fatting Oils

Super fatting in soap making is sometimes called **lye discounting**, which means that a soap maker can either add extra oil to a soap recipe while keeping the amount of lye the same, or reduce the amount of lye in the soap recipe while keeping the amount of oil the same. Super fatting oils are high in fatty acids and help produce soaps that are moisturizing. They should be added to your soap recipe at trace after all your other ingredients, already mixed in with lye, have started to thicken and are less likely to separate from each other. Adding the super fatting oils at this stage prevents them from reacting to the caustic lye, which often changes chemical compositions of oils, making them less therapeutic.

Apricot kernel

Some soap makers refer to apricot kernel as the perfect all-around oil that can be used for all types of skin types, while being gentle as needed or giving a little extra strength if needed as well. As a super fatting oil, it can help repair dehydrated, sensitive, or prematurely aging skin. For soap making, use it at 10 percent in combination with coconut oil, olive oil, and palm oil.

Argan

Though still more of an unknown oil in the aromatherapy field, argan oil gets high marks from those who use it because of its reputation for having great anti-aging properties and for being a lightweight oil that is rich in essential fatty acids and vitamin E. It comes from the seeds of the heavily protected argan tree (*argania spinosa*), which is native to Morocco. The oil retails for about $15 to $30 per fluid ounce, making it very expensive and a good candidate to blend with other, less costly base oils.

Argan oil is used for cooking, as well as cosmetic and therapeutic benefits. These benefits and its price make it a good candidate for use in super fatting soap. Blend it at less than 30 percent with jojoba for a moisturizing soap, and blend with tea tree for soap that treats skin conditions such as acne, eczema, psoriasis, stretch marks, and sunburns. Argan oil soap is soft with creamy, stable lather.

Babassu

Cold pressed from the kernels of the Amazon native babassu palm trees (*orbignya phalerata*), this oil is a white solid at room temperature and a very effective emollient when used to super fatten soaps. It is very similar to coconut and palm kernel oils in that it can dry the soap if used at more than 30 percent. Babassu oil soap is hard with full lather and plenty of suds.

Black cumin

This oil is cold pressed from the seeds of the *nigella sativa*, an herb native to Egypt and Turkey and used for culinary, cosmetic, and therapeutic purposes. It is considered a panacea for therapeutic purposes, because it can help with a wide range of problems, internally and externally, including as an antibacterial, antihistamine, and pain reliever. For soap making, use it in equal parts combination with shea butter and jojoba. It produces a soft, dark-colored, herbal scented soap.

Borage

When used to super fatten soap, borage oil retains its therapeutic properties and can help fend off dry skin, sun damage, eczema, and other skin conditions. Borage oil is a powerful emollient and produces a slightly hard soap with good, stable lather. Use at no more than 10 percent in your oils batch.

Brazil nut

The oil expressed from the *bertholletia excelsa* tree native to Brazil is emollient and can be used for cosmetic and for therapeutic purposes, including for the treatment of skin conditions such as eczema and psoriasis. It is rich in proteins and vitamins A and E. Its recommended use in soap making should be at 5 percent in combination with olive or castor oil.

Castor

Castor oil (*ricinus communis*) attracts and retains moisture in the skin. It can be used alone or in combination with other oils like coconut or aloe. Used alone, it results in a soft, transparent soap with thick lather. For harder soap, use it at 20 percent in combination with other oils like coconut.

Emu oil

Emu oil, from the fat of the emu bird, is often referred to as nature's finest emollient because of its high levels of fatty acids that make it an excellent moisturizer and skin softener that is not greasy, does not clog pores, and is highly penetrating. It is said to promote faster healing of burns with minimal scarring as well as acting as an anti-inflammatory. Use at up to 10 percent with olive oil and sunflower oil for a mild soap with stable lather.

Evening primrose

Evening primrose oil is extracted from *oenothera biennis*, a small, yellow wildflower now cultivated just for oil production. The oil, unlike all the other oils covered in this chapter, is a good source of essential fatty acids, a group of rare acids more commonly known as vitamin F. Used as a super fattening soap oil, evening primrose oil can restore elasticity to mature skin, reducing wrinkles, and reduce dryness. The soap is soft and mild and has good, stable lather. Use at 5 to 10 percent with hempseed oil and olive oil.

Grapeseed

Grapeseed oil should be used at 5 percent with avocado oil, castor oil, cocoa butter, and apricot kernel oil. It has powerful antioxidant and astringent properties that protect skin cells while moisturizing and toning. It produces a mild, soft soap with stable lather.

Flaxseed

Flaxseed oil is cold pressed from the seeds of *linum usitatissimum*, an herbaceous annual plant that can be found in most parts of the world. The oil in super fattened soap is super moisturizing and can help improve skin conditions like acne, eczema, psoriasis, and soften dry and mature skin. It is an inflammatory that can heal burns, cuts, and reduce the appearance of rashes. It has a short shelf life — three months — so use should be capped at 5 percent to prevent the soap from going bad quickly. Use with olive oil and sweet almond oil for a soft and mild soap. Add coconut, castor, or palm kernel oils for bubbly lather.

Hazelnut

Hazelnut oil has astringent properties and high content of essential fatty acids that help tone the skin while moisturizing dry and mature skin. Use it at up to 10 percent with grapeseed oil for a good conditioning and soft soap.

Jojoba

Jojoba is more of a liquid wax than an oil and is an excellent and nourishing moisturizer for extra dry skin. Use it at 5 percent to super fatten soap made with castor and sunflower oil.

Lanolin

Sometimes called wool fat, lanolin is the oily wax found on the skin of sheep and is released when sheep are sheered and separated from their wool. This heavy wax oil attracts moisture and is absorbed within the skin, making it good for dry skin and perfect for super fattening soap. It produces soft, mild soap with stable, creamy lather. Use at 5 percent with olive and coconut oil.

Mango butter

Mango butter is cold pressed from the seed kernel of the *mangifera indica*, a tropical tree. It is a solid at room temperature, is a wonderful emollient, and is very useful in moisturizing and softening the skin. When used as a super fatting oil, at about 5 to 15 percent, mango butter results in a rich, smooth soap. It can be substituted for shea butter.

Neem

Neem oil is cold pressed from the whole nuts of the *azadirachta indica* tree. It is a magnificent oil that traces quickly and has antibacterial, antifungal, antiseptic, and antiviral properties. When used to super fatten soap, neem oil's antiseptic properties are useful in the treatment of dandruff. It can also be used in liquid soap to repel insects when sprayed on plant leaves.

Ostrich

This very moisturizing oil, as the name suggests, comes from the fat of the ostrich, which is rendered for use in balms, creams, and soaps. Ostrich oil, when used as a super fatting oil, retains properties that make it useful in the treatment of burns, dry skin, eczema, psoriasis, and other ailments for thousands of years. Although it is a rich oil, it does not clog pores, meaning that it is noncomedogenic. Use with mango butter and olive oil at up to 15 percent of your total oil batch for a soft, creamy soap.

Pistachio

Pistachio oil is cold pressed from the pistachio nut. It is high in unsaturated fatty acids and vitamin E, making it excellent for hydrating and moisturizing the skin. You can use this oil at about 6 percent of your total oils. It is an excellent emollient oil that nourishes and softens the skin without leaving a greasy feeling. It absorbs rapidly, making it excellent in all skin care products, lip balms, body sprays, and bath oils. Use this oil together with sweet almond, coconut, and olive oil.

Pumpkin seed

Pumpkin seed oil absorbs well into the skin; is rich in vitamins A, E, C, and K; and helps the skin regenerate by healing scars, slowing aging, and soothing other skin conditions, including dryness. Use at no more than 3 percent in combination with hemp seed oil for a soft, stable soap.

Rosehip

Rosehip oil is rich in fatty acids and when used as a super fattening oil, can work wonders on the skin. It can help the skin regenerate faster, which means that it helps minimize the appearance of scars and the effects of aging. The oil can be used as a coloring agent because of its pink color. Use up to 10 percent in combination with coconut oil, olive oil, and palm oil for a soft soap with stable lather.

Shea butter

Shea butter comes from the fruit pits of the African butter tree. It is a popular oil/fat because of its moisturizing and nourishing abilities. The fact that it is easily available and quite economical also adds to its appeal. As a super fattening soap oil, shea butter provides the skin with the benefits of essential fatty acids and vitamins A, E, and F. The latter of these softens the skin by keeping dryness at bay and retaining moisture in the skin. It also helps regenerate the skin. It produces a hard, mild soap with stable and creamy lather. Use at up to 30 percent with castor oil for more bubbly lather.

Sweet almond

Sweet almond oil is an easy oil to use when making soap because it traces quickly, producing a mild soap with creamy and stable lather. It is rather expensive, hence its use as a super fatting oil. Use at up to 10 percent with oils that have longer shelf lives that can lengthen its short shelf life. Use with calendula and jojoba for a moisturizing bar with creamy lather.

Walnut oil

Walnut oil is very emollient, deeply penetrating, and very good for use on dry, cracked, and otherwise damaged skin. It is slow to trace but can be used at 10 percent with olive oil and palm oil for slightly faster trace and longer shelf life of more than three months. Walnut oil produces a soft, good conditioning soap with stable lather.

Other Nutrients

The beauty and uniqueness of homemade soap is in the sheer artistry and the many possible infusions you can add to the soap to make its properties and textures more appealing to you, allowing you to choose when you can use a smooth soap or a scrubby soap. Adding spices, herbs, botanicals, and organics to your soap can also add to its scent, color, and therapeutic benefits. The following represent some of the additional elements you can add to your soaps to create a personalized aromatherapy soap.

Herbs

There are numerous herbs, dried or fresh, that can enhance your soap. Basil, paprika, parsley, rosemary, and thyme can be ground, chopped into small pieces, or used whole in soap making. They can be added to the saponified soap mixture just before it is poured into molds or they can be added to the water or oils your recipe calls for.

Exfoliants

Exfoliants are additives that give your soap a bit of a rough texture and scrubbing power. They include flower petals, herbs, peels, seeds, spices, and other items that work best when ground to fine powder and added at trace. They are useful for scrubbing away dead skin, leaving the skin soft and supple. In addition to their use as exfoliants, these additives can add a different dimension to the nutrient level, color, and aroma in your soap.

Honey and beeswax

Sweet smelling soap is one of the advantages of using honey and beeswax in your soap. The high sugar content in honey creates a great, creamy lather, and both honey and beeswax are great for moisturizing your skin because they are humectants that draw and retain moisture. Experienced soap makers, when using honey and beeswax in their recipes, love to use a hive or bee mold for an aesthetically pleasing product.

Honey and beeswax recipe

To make a honey and beeswax soap, try the following recipe.

INGREDIENTS

1 Tbsp. honey

1 Tbsp. beeswax

1 cup unscented glycerin soap base

Dash of bee pollen, if desired

DIRECTIONS

1. Melt beeswax in double boiler. Remember, equipment and utensils used for soap making can no longer be used in food preparation.

2. Mix beeswax with the melted soap base.

3. Add honey and stir until melted.

4. Add bee pollen, if desired.

5. Carefully pour your soap into the mold, preferably wearing gloves to protect your hands.

6. Release the soap from the mold when it has completely hardened.

7. Let your homemade beeswax soap cure on a drying rack.

Clays

You may rarely think of clay as a promoter of health but clay has promoted health in plants, animals, and humans for centuries, if not since the beginning of time. Clay can be used to treat internal and external ailments such as the flu, hemorrhoids, ulcers, viral infections, acne, and open wounds. Clay, said to carry a negative electrical charge, has also been used in battling food poisoning, toxins, and other impurities by attracting to the positive charges these impurities carry.

Soap makers can use many types of clay in soap making but there are four clay types that are most popular, all with interchangeable functions. They include:

- **Bentonite** – also called montmorillonite, it is a highly absorbent green clay used in many applications, including cosmetically in face masks

- **Kaolin** – sometimes referred to as white cosmetic clay due to its color, it is found in powdered cosmetics

- **Rhassoul** – called red clay, it is actually brown in color and is used for exfoliating

- **Rose clay** – closely related to kaolin, it is used mostly for its rose color that comes from iron oxides but can also add to soap's absorbency

Organics

Why put organics like fruits and vegetables in soap? Could they rot and spoil the soap? The simple answer is that these organics are rich in nutrients, vitamins, and enzymes that are good for the body. They can also enhance the aesthetics and fragrance of the soap. They are used in forms, such as powder, that do not encourage rotting. That said, you can use the following organic items in any of your homemade soaps:

- **Fruits and vegetables:** These can be pureed or dried and crushed to powder form for use in your soaps. Popular botanicals include bananas, carrots, cucumbers, mangoes, pumpkins, and strawberries.

- **Eggs:** Protein rich and emollient, you can add eggs to a basic soap ingredient at trace. One egg is enough for a 2-pound batch of soap with smaller batches requiring just a fraction of an egg.

Seaweed

You do not have to go deep sea diving to find these nutrient-rich weeds. Laden with minerals such as iodine and iron and trace elements like boron, chromium, and zinc, seaweed is said to be able to penetrate the skin's subcutaneous layer and

• • •

reduce the accumulation of fat, thereby leading to a leaner body. In soap making, seaweed can be used fresh, powdered, in flakes, or as an extract. Fresh seaweed is readily available in whole foods markets where you can find sushi ingredients.

Silk

Silk is synonymous with luxury and even self-indulgence. Different kinds of silk products derived from the cocoon of the domesticated silkworm are used to create silky soap. These products, after a refining process to remove impurities, include silk amino acids, silk fiber, silk powder, and hydrolyzed silk and are available from soap supply, fiber art, and online stores. They are mostly imported from China.

- **Silk amino acids** include 18 kinds of amino acids. These are molecules made out of amino and carboxylic acids and are essential for various nutritional values, including protein and energy. These amino acids are quickly absorbed into the skin and can nourish and repair damaged skin cells.

- **Silk fiber** can be added to your soap-making water before or after you add lye, with the latter being the more preferred method. The fibers dissolve in the hot lye mixture for a silky bar that provides shine and elasticity to the skin.

- **Silk powder**, like silk fiber, can be added before or after the addition of lye.

- **Hydrolyzed silk** has been subjected to alkali to produce water-soluble silk protein that is easily absorbed into the skin and helpful in moisture retention to avoid dry skin. It should be added at no more than 2 percent of your total soap solution ingredients.

Aloe vera

Aloe vera is extracted from the *aloe barbadensis miller*, an African native short-stemmed plant of the same name. The plant, nicknamed the "miracle plant," thrives in hot weather and is a popular houseplant because of its versatility as a healer, ingredient in cosmetics, and culinary ingredient. Its lower leaf, when sliced open, releases a gel that is used for medicinal purposes to detoxify the body, heal burns, treat other skin conditions, and act as an antibacterial, among other things.

Preservatives

Natural soap makers do not rely on synthetic preservatives to lengthen the shelf lives of their products. The alkali in homemade soap helps inhibit bacteria, yeast, and mold growth. They are most common in super fattened soaps and those made using oils with shorter shelf lives.

If you choose to keep all your soap ingredients natural, try to incorporate oil like rosemary in your soap, because it has a shelf life of up to four years. Beyond that, to keep your soap fresh, use fresh ingredients and clean equipment; store soaps in a cool, dry place; and avoid plastic storage containers that trap moisture inside the soap.

Color

Color makes soap more appealing to the eye and can be one of the more fun parts of creating soap, giving you a chance to satisfy the sense of artistry you may have. Coloring your soap is best attempted once you have successfully made several batches of soap and feel comfortable with the soap-making process. You might be interested in creating a soap coloring that matches a particular scent (for example, lavender for lavender-scented soap), is as orange as the sky at sunset, or is a mixture of two or more favorite shades. There is a kaleidoscope of colors that you can use to make your soap visually appealing, some synthetic and some natural.

Synthetic versus natural

Natural colorants are plant based or mineral based and are often less likely to cause adverse reactions like itching or inflammation to the skin, especially when used in small quantities required in soap making. Still, some natural colorants can be irritating to the skin and others like iron oxide, which is mined from earth, have very high levels of heavy metals such as lead and mercury that have been found to be dangerous to humans and animals. Mercury can cause cancer and lead can result in less mental acuity in children.

Synthetic colorants, also called FD and C (food, drug, and cosmetic) colors, can be useful and less expensive. The drawback in using them is that the laboratory chemistry that produces these synthetic dyes and pigments can cause some irritation. The best rule of thumb to use when considering colorants is to do your homework. Find out the pros and cons of each colorant with special emphasis on their effects on your and your family's health and well-being.

Types of coloring agents

The four main types of colorants are botanical (plant based), dyes, micas (minerals), and pigments.

Plant Oils, Vegetable Compounds, and Plant Extracts

Each part of a plant can contribute to the color pallet. The roots, barks, leaves, fruits, and essential oils of many plants bear color, but whether the color can be used in soap depends upon several factors, such as, how efficient it is to extract the color? And, how they react in lye, heat, or cold?

Minerals

Also called micas, minerals are derived from the earth by mining and include several varieties of iron oxides in several colors including black, blue, brown, green, pink, red, and yellow. They are mostly available in powder form and can be used in cold processing, a method of soap making that requires no heat; hot processing, which requires heat; and the melt and pour method, which involves melting a glycerin soap base, using additives, and pouring into a mold. A test using a small amount of micas in your soap mixture can help and is recommended to determine how the color reacts to lye and whether the final hue appeals to you.

Dyes

Soap dyes can be either natural or synthetic, powdered or liquid. To use them properly, infuse them with a small portion of the super fatting oil you will be using in your recipe and add at trace. Remember that lye can alter natural dye colors, making the final color very unlike what you might have expected. Synthetic dyes, also called pigment, tend to be more consistent.

Pigments

These were originally from ultramarines (deep blue pigments) and oxides from mineral sources like clay and sodium carbonate but the FDA deemed them unsafe, thereby opening a market for the synthetic recreation. They are very stable in soap making, meaning they do not bleed and hardly react with lye. When using them, mix thoroughly to avoid clumping.

Fragrance

Adding your favorite scent to your homemade soap just serves to enhance it even more. The most common fragrance to add to your soap is from essential oils and synthetic fragrance oils, which are not recommended if you want your soap to be therapeutic. Both essential oils and synthetic fragrance oils are usually added at trace, drop-by-drop in conservative quantities, so they do not "seize" your soap. Seized soap takes on the texture of mashed potatoes and may need to be discarded.

Adding fragrance to soaps

The drop-by-drop method of adding essential and fragrance oils can be substituted by infusing the scents in the water or base oils you seek to use in your soap mixture. For instance, you can infuse the scent of chamomile in your soap. To infuse the scent of chamomile, you would have to steep chamomile petals in the water you will use in soap making for at least 30 minutes.

Choosing fragrances

Each nose likes what it likes; therefore, choosing fragrance is a very subjective process. If using essential oils, remember how notes blend with each other. Take that into consideration when choosing fragrance for your soap.

Essential Oils Versus Fragrance Oils

Essential oils come from all natural ingredients while fragrance oils are a combination of natural ingredients and synthetic ingredients. In aromatherapy, all natural ingredients are always preferred over synthetic ingredients. Avoid oils that could be sensitizing to you and never use toxic oils.

Armed with the knowledge of what soap is and what is needed to make soap, you can now better understand the different methods of soap making. The following chapter covers these methods as well as fancy yet simple techniques to make homemade soap appealing to the eye.

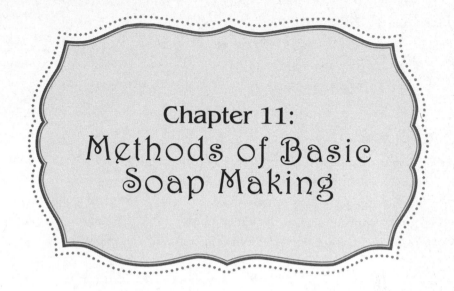

Chapter 11:
Methods of Basic Soap Making

Soap makers describe the overall process of soap making as science meeting art. And just as there are different methods of painting, there are different methods of soap making. The distinguishing factors in these methods are heat, or the lack of it, and a few other key points discussed below. *Recipes are provided in Chapter 12.*

Cold Process

This is the earliest form and most popular method; the one grandma used. The only heat necessary for this process is the heat created when lye dissolves in water, and the heat required to melt any solid fats a soap-making recipe calls for. Soap making requires exceptional detail to lye measurements but even more so when using the cold process method. Lye becomes less active and less caustic faster in hot process soaps than in cold process soaps, which typically have to cure for weeks to achieve the same lye effect. It is best to study the saponification chart for the saponification value of fats and oils being used so as to calculate the appropriate amount of lye to use. *This chart is included in Chapter 15.*

Benefits of method

Making soap this way can be very rewarding, because you have control over everything that goes into your soap. Additionally, soap made this way is more economical in the long run than soap made using the hot process method.

Getting started

Have all your equipment and ingredients within reach before you begin making your soap. Line your wooden molds with freezer paper or spray your plastic mold with vegetable oil spray. Don your apron, gloves, and goggles and make sure you are in a well ventilated area to allow the fumes from the lye solution to quickly dissipate. A nice, flat working surface in your backyard is even better.

Directions

1. Measure the lye and its container on a scale.

2. Measure the water the same way.

3. In a well ventilated area and using a heat resistant container, mix the lye and water by slowly adding the lye to the water. Never mix them by adding the water to the lye to avoid a volcanic-type explosive reaction.

4. Stir the mixture carefully for several minutes until the lye dissolves and the water is clear. This mixture can get to be at hot as 200 degrees, so be very careful.

5. Place the lye solution in a bucket of ice to cool, aiming for a temperature of 92 to 100 degrees.

6. Measure and melt any solid oils and fats you have for your recipe at a low heat. Once they are melted, mix them with your liquid oils. Check the temperature to ensure it is between 92 and 100 degrees. Use the bucket of ice to cool them if necessary.

7. Pour the cooled lye solution into the oils, stirring gently to avoid splashing the caustic solution. You can use plastic coverings to cover your work surface for an extra layer of protection. For faster results, use a stick blender on the mixture until trace begins to appear and the mixture thickens.

8. Measure and add any other nutrients — herbs, essential oils, super fatting oils — your recipe calls for.

9. Make sure every ingredient is mixed-in properly then pour it into the mold, using a plastic spatula to scrape any remnants.

10. Cover the mold and insulate it with some bath towels. Let it sit uninterrupted for at least 24 hours, until it is firm enough for you to make gentle impressions with your finger. Cut off any residue or white speckles on top of the soap.

11. Cut the soap into manageable bars and let it sit or cure for at least four weeks before use. The soap becomes milder the longer it cures.

Hot Process

This process only differs from the cold process method because the soap mixture is cooked before being placed in a mold. This speeds up the curing process and instead of needing the soap to cure for a few days or weeks, it only needs to cure for a few hours.

Benefits of method

Because your wait time is cut by more than half, you can use your beautiful homemade soap sooner than if you use the cold process method. Another benefit is that once the lye solution and oils mixture has cooked, the lye is completely neutralized prior to the addition of essential oils for fragrance and other additives. This ensures the essential oils used to add fragrance to the soap do not evaporate during a lengthy curing process and they maintain their therapeutic properties.

Getting started

Set up by readying all your equipment and ingredients by placing them within reach of your work station. Line your wooden molds with freezer paper or spray your plastic mold with vegetable oil spray. Don your apron, gloves, and goggles and make sure you are in a well ventilated area to allow the fumes from the lye solution to quickly dissipate. Additionally, make sure you either have a slow cooker or a pre-heated oven ready to cook the soap.

Directions

1. Measure the lye and its container on a scale.

2. Measure the water the same way.

3. In a well ventilated area and using a heat resistant container, mix the lye and water by slowly adding the lye to the water. Never mix them by adding the water to the lye to avoid a volcanic-type explosion.

4. Stir the mixture carefully for several minutes until the lye dissolves and the water is clear. This mixture can get to be at hot as 200 degrees, so be very careful.

5. Place the lye solution in a bucket of ice to cool, aiming for a temperature of 92 to 100 degrees.

6. Measure and melt any solid oils and fats you have for your recipe at a low heat. Once they are melted, mix them with your liquid oils. Check the temperature to ensure it is between 92 and 100 degrees. Use the bucket of ice to cool them if necessary.

7. Pour your lye solution and oils blend into a slow cooker at 160 degrees and use a stick blender to help bring it to trace.

8. Once it gets to trace, cover the mixture and let it cook for ten minutes. Stir the mixture and if the edges are flaking, mix them in with the rest of the batch. Let it cook, stirring it every ten minutes until the mixture begins to look like mashed potatoes and it can no longer "zap" or sting you the way a 9 volt battery would. This means the lye has neutralized and is no longer caustic. You can also cook the mixture in an oven at 160 degrees, stirring every 15 minutes. The mixture can be ready in as little as 45 minutes to two hours.

9. Add your nutrients, fragrance, super fatting oil, and color if your recipe is incorporating them.

10. Scoop the cooked, goopy mixture into your mold and tap the mold firmly on the counter to get rid of any air pockets.

11. Cover the top of the soap with a plastic wrap and press the top with your fingers to smooth it out.

12. Allow it to cool down to room temperature then remove from mold.

13. Cut and use as soon as the soap is firm enough.

Milk Soaps

Using milk in any recipe, culinary or otherwise, is a promise that the final product will be rich, creamy, and decadent. In soap making, goat's milk is popular mainly because of label appeal, but cow's milk and coconut milk are also used. Some soap makers use powdered milk, but this is not recommended in aromatherapy because of the synthetic preservatives found in this type of milk. When making milk-based soaps, it is important to understand that milk has sugar, which can caramelize in hot temperatures and turn the final product brown.

Benefits of method

Using milk creates a wonderfully emollient and nutritious soap that is beneficial to the skin. Peptides in the milk encourage collagen development, leading to more elastic and younger looking skin.

Getting started

Set up just like you would when using the cold process method and place all your safety and measuring equipment within reach of your workstation. When using fresh milk, you can either pasteurize it beforehand by boiling it at 155 degrees or use it as is, letting the chemical reaction that occurs when you mix the lye into the milk do the trick. Pasteurization kills any harmful organisms like bacteria that can be found in animal products.

Directions

1. Measure lye and its container on a scale.

2. Measure milk the same way.

3. In a well ventilated area and using a heat resistant container, mix the lye and milk by slowly adding the lye to the milk. Never mix them by adding the milk to the lye to avoid a volcanic-type reaction. For better results, place the milk in a tub of ice and slowly add the lye. This helps prevent rapid caramelization or curdling, because it reduces the temperature of the mixture. Caramelization and curdling can spoil your soap by giving it a burnt smell and uneven texture.

4. Stir the mixture carefully for several minutes until the lye dissolves and the water is clear. This mixture can get to be at hot as 200 degrees so be very careful.

5. Place the lye solution in a bucket of ice to cool, aiming for a temperature of 92 to 100 degrees.

6. Measure and melt any solid oils and fats you have for your recipe at a low heat. Once they are melted, mix them with your liquid oils. Check the temperature to ensure it is between 92 and 100 degrees.

7. Pour the cooled lye solution into the oils, stirring gently to avoid splashing the caustic solution. You can use plastic coverings to cover your work surface for additional protection as well. For faster results, use a stick blender on the mixture until trace begins to appear and the mixture thickens.

8. Measure and add any other nutrients, herbs, essential oils, and super fatting oils your recipe calls for.

9. Follow the steps in the cold process method but substitute water with milk in your lye solution. Transfer the mixture into molds and cover. The mixture does not require extra insulation by being covered with bath towels once it is placed in molds, because it remains warm for a longer period.

10. Make sure to let the soap cure four to six weeks before use. This is very important to prevent the soap from dissolving too fast when used.

11. You can also make milk soap using the hot process but substituting the milk for the water.

Basic Soap Recipe

INGREDIENTS

12 ounces cold distilled water

4.2 ounces lye

4 ounces tallow

12 ounces castor oil

12 ounces olive or canola oil

4 ounces palm kernel oil

DIRECTIONS

1. Weigh all your ingredients and set them aside.

2. In a well-ventilated area, and with all your safety equipment set and ready, using a heat resistant container, slowly add the lye to the water, stirring the mixture thoroughly. Do this with caution because the mixture can get very hot.

3. Melt your saturated fat and mix it with the other oils — castor, olive, canola, and palm kernel oils.

4. Allow the oils and the lye solution to cool to no more than 100 degrees.

5. Add the lye solution to the oils, stirring thoroughly.

6. Keep stirring vigorously for about ten minutes until the mixture thickens. A stick blender can be useful at this stage.

7. Pour mixture into soap molds, cover with bath towels, and let sit for 24 hours.

8. Your soap will be ready to use after it cures in about three weeks. Letting the soap sit in room temperatures to cure allows soap to become mild and allows extra water to evaporate.

This recipe makes about 2 pounds of soap but can be adjusted depending on your need. Note that it is always a good idea to start small, because this allows you to make mistakes without using many ingredients.

Hand Milling

This process is also called the "rebatch method" and involves reprocessing previously made soap, either from your own kitchen, another soap maker, or from a wholesale supplier. It allows you to reuse soap that might not have come out as you wanted, giving you a second chance to fix bad color or find a use for ugly soap.

Benefits of method

The hand milling method is very time-friendly because it requires no more than an hour to make a ready-to-use soap bar. It requires no safety equipment like goggles and gloves because you are not using caustic lye. Finally, this method produces soap that lasts longer than other homemade or commercially available soaps so it is very economical.

Getting started

Using this method requires just a knife to cut the soap base, a slow cooker or double boiler to melt glycerin soap base, and a pre-lined or pre-greased soap mold. You should also measure out and prepare additives like coloring, essential oils, exfoliants, and herbs.

Directions

1. Cut or grate the pre-made soap into bite-size pieces.
2. Use a slow cooker or a double boiler to melt the glycerin soap base.
3. Once the base is melted, add your choice of additives such as herbs and color.
4. Pour the resulting product into the readied mold. Work quickly so the soap does not get too hard and become difficult to pour into the mold.
5. Once in the mold, let the soap cool for one or more hours then cut and use.

Liquid Soaps

Liquid soaps require using potassium hydroxide as opposed to lye in powder form or as a sodium hydroxide solution. The molecules in the potassium hydroxide are said to be larger, which enables the resulting soap to maintain a liquid state. Alternately, you can make liquid soap by taking one of your hard bar soaps, adding honey, glycerin, and water to make liquid soap or making castile soap, which is just saponified olive oil and water.

Benefits of method

This soap-making method produces soap that lathers well and is very easy to use. Castile liquid soap, like other natural soaps, is a good alternative to harsh liquid detergents in the market.

Getting started

Ready all the equipment and ingredients you would normally use for the hot process method. Set up by readying all your equipment and ingredients and placing them within reach of your work station. Line your wooden molds with freezer paper or spray your plastic mold with vegetable oil spray. Don your apron, gloves, and goggles and make sure you are in a well ventilated area to allow the fumes from the lye solution to dissipate quickly. Additionally, make sure you either have a slow cooker or a pre-heated oven ready to cook the soap.

Note that liquid soap recipes call for about 10 percent "lye excess" and some boric acid, which you can purchase from supermarkets, to neutralize the mixture after it has cooked. You will also need a large glass bottle, at least 40 ounces, with a lid and plenty of patience because the process required to make liquid soap is more complicated than the basic hot process.

Directions

1. Measure out your oils and place them in a slow cooker.
2. Mix your potassium hydroxide into water carefully and stir until it becomes clear. Let it cool in an ice bucket until it reaches about 100 degrees.

3. Add the lye solution to your oils, stirring it for a minute or two.

4. Introduce the stick blender and use until trace begins. This can take up to 30 minutes depending on the oils you are using.

5. Once it gets to trace, make sure the temperature is at 160 degrees. Cover the slow cooker and check on it every 15 to 30 minutes, making sure to stir it well each time. There are times when the mixture gets very tough but stir it the best you can, using a potato masher if necessary.

6. This process can take up to four hours. You will know your soap mixture is ready when the mixture looks like translucent petroleum jelly. To be sure it is ready, dissolve 1 ounce of the soap mixture into 2 ounces of boiling water. If it is milky or very cloudy, it is not ready. If it is clear or just a bit cloudy and stays that way even after it cools, then it is ready. Once the soap mixture is ready, dissolve the rest of the mixture into the same water ratio.

7. Cover the mixture and let it sit for about an hour. Stir it after each hour. You can also let it sit and soften overnight then use the potato masher to break it up.

8. Once the mixture is completely dissolved, turn on the slow cooker at 180 degrees.

9. Dissolve the boric acid in very hot water. You need about a ¾ ounce of this neutralizing solution for every pound of soap mixture you have.

10. While the neutralizing solution is still very hot, pour it 1 ounce at a time into the slow cooker soap mixture and stir well, removing any cloudiness. A warm or cold solution will not dissolve in your soap mixture because the boric acid precipitates out of the solution as it cools.

11. Now you can add colorants, fragrance, and other additives and mix well.

12. Transfer this mixture from the slow cooker to a large bottle with a lid and let it sit where it cannot be disturbed, ensuring the mixture remains at room temperature. This is called **sequestering**. After three weeks, you can transfer the resultant liquid soap into the final bottles. Try not to disturb any insoluble particles that form from your ingredients at the bottom of the large bottle. If necessary, use a sieve and throw away these particles.

Melt and Pour

This is the method used to make clear soap. It is a very simple process that lasts just about 15 minutes from beginning to end. The melt and pour method involves melting a pre-made clear glycerin base, available from craft stores and from natural soap makers, and being creative with color and fragrance. Glycerin base is a mixture of vegetable oils and glycerin.

Benefits of method

This is a very simple way to make soap. Glycerin-based soap creates a more moisturizing product that is very gentle and cleansing.

Getting started

You need a slow cooker, double boiler, or microwave to melt your soap base. You also need a pre-lined or pre-greased mold and a whisk to stir the base when needed to make sure it is completely melted.

Directions

1. Melt the soap base.
2. Add any other ingredients you desire, like colorants, fragrance, herbs, and decorations like swirls.
3. Place in the mold and allow it to firm up.
4. Use immediately if so desired.

Fancy Techniques

The sky is the limit if you choose to add fancy techniques to your soap making. Soap makers who use fancy techniques are artists of a different level than regular soap makers. The inspiration often comes from food, especially desserts. Swirling and marbling are the most common soap decorative techniques available. Others include layering and chunking and they can all be employed using any of the soap making methods already discussed.

Swirling and marbling

Swirling involves using two or more colors in your soap in a way that makes it look like it has swirls in it. This is achieved by finding the perfect consistency of your soap mixture right at trace — it should neither be too thin nor too thick. Transfer your soap into the mold and add your fragrances and other additives.

Next, you can add color by pouring in one color at a time. Hold your color container high and away from the mold if you want your swirls to get to the bottom of the soap mixture. Lower it and pour the color closer to the mold if you want the swirls to be superficial and stay on top of the soaps mixture. Run a chopstick once or twice to spread the color around then let your soap set and firm up before cutting it.

For marbling, do not pour all your soap mixture into the mold but rather hold it back so you can add color to it while it is still in the pot. When the color is to your liking, gently add the mixture to the mold. This process gives the soap a marbled look when it firms up and is cut.

Layering

With layering, you can get the benefit of two or more scents, two colors, or two textures in one soap. Layering requires dividing up your soap batch at light trace just before adding color and other additives. Use a heat-resistant glass container to help you measure the batches, keeping the amount of each batch as equal to the other as possible. Once divided, you can add whatever additives and color you desire to each individual batch. Be careful to measure your additions with the consideration that you are working with two half batches instead of one full batch.

Pour the first batch into a mold followed by the second batch once it is ready. Do not pour the second batch too fast if you want to avoid a swirling effect. Cover and insulate the mold and let it sit for 24 hours until it is firm and you can make gentle impressions with your fingers. Cut it and let it cure four to six weeks.

Chunking

This allows you to add small pieces of colorful soap to your bar and lets creativity reign. If you are using the melt and pour method, cut, cover with plastic wrap, and melt clear glycerin soap base in a microwave for about 30 seconds. Stir the base and pop it back in the microwave for a few more seconds if solid chunks still exist. Add additives and separate the now liquid base into half with one half going into several small bowls — depending on how many colors you want to use — and the other half for use as "background base." Add colorants to each bowl.

Pour some background base into a mold, and tap it hard to get rid of air bubbles. Some soap makers use isopropyl alcohol to get rid of air bubbles. Pour several thin layers of the colored bases on a piece of freezer paper and allow it to cool then chop it into chunky pieces and scatter them over the background base. You can make a second, third, or fourth layer using the same process before finishing off with the background base. Allow the resulting product to sit and firm up for 24 hours before cutting and enjoying your colorful creation. This technique can also be employed for cold or hot process soaps with chunk pieces added at trace with other additives.

Embossing

Embossing soap is like putting your own unique stamp on it. You can emboss soap made using the cold process, hot process, hand milling, or melt and pour methods using embossers available at craft stores. You can even order specially made embossers with your name or logo, if you are planning to sell your soaps.

To emboss, wait a day or two after cutting your soap just to give it breathing room. Your soap is still soft enough to take on a stamp easily. Use a small mallet to tap the embosser a few times into each bar of soap. Remove any loose pieces using a soft, unused toothbrush or a tissue. You may need a few practice runs before you get the feel of the process, but you will love seeing your stamp on the final product.

Embedding

The embedding method is like stuffing your soap and works easier with melt and pour soap, because you can often use individual bar soap molds, which make the embedding process easier. However, you can also use the embedding method when making soaps using other methods. After melting your glycerin base, pour it into your molds about three quarters of the way full to leave room for your embedding objects, which you can then add and allow to firm up with the soap. If your soap is made using any other method, you can always add embedding objects when you are adding your additives like herbs and colorants.

Embedding objects are available at craft stores and can be geometric shapes, shapes of little things found in nature, and other fun objects like plastic insects.

Troubleshooting

There are several minute things that can spoil the perfect batch of soap you envisioned. Common problems with appearance and texture, among other things, may develop from using impure ingredients, incorrect measurements, or the wrong additives. Soap making is very much a trial and error process and taking notes of what you do each time you make a batch will help you keep track of what you do right or wrong. Some major problems involve incorrect lye amounts but these can be easily avoided by using a handy online lye calculator, careful calculations, and strict adherence to recipes.

Appearance problems

- If your soap has a bit of white ash on top, it may just mean that the lye cooled too fast. Use a pH strip to test alkalinity and make sure the white ash is not lye. A pH value of 7 is safe and all you need to do to fix this minor problem is to cut away the white substance.

- Sometimes soap can have too many air bubbles. This means that it was stirred too long and though it may not look perfect, you can still use it.

- If your soap is cracked, irregular looking, or the color is not what you expected, you can reuse it in another batch or use it as is.

Texture problems

- If the soap is too grainy or too hard, it may be seized soap. Seized soap looks like chunky, dried up mashed potatoes instead of a smoother version. Rebatching this soap can help.

- Soap that will not trace may have too little lye but using a stick blender for up to three hours with breaks in between may speed up trace. If it still does not trace, let it sit for 24 hours. If this does not help, discard the mixture.

When to throw your soap away

You will know you need to throw your soap away when any of the following happens:

- When soap is too hard and crumbles when cut, there is too much lye.

- When soap is too soft and spongy after two weeks of curing, there is too much lye, water, or oils. Take good notes and recalculate your measurements to prevent this from happening again.

- When there are lye pockets in the soap.

- Where there is more than a little white ash on top, covering every top part of the soap, this means the water used was too hard or the lye did not dissolve.

- When the soap oozes a liquid when cut, this could be lye that did not saponify and is still caustic.

- When the soap separates in the mold and there is a greasy layer on top of a hard soap, this means there was not enough lye or the mixture was not stirred enough.

CASE STUDY: DELORES DEAN

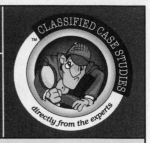

Richmond, Va.
Delores Dean, a nurse by profession, who started dabbling in aromatherapy in the 1970s.

"That was a time for awakening," she said. "I wanted to know what was going on and two things appealed to me — religion and natural body care. I started reading the ingredient labels on every product I used and I wanted to know where I could find the ingredients so I visited earth shops, shows, and other places so I could learn, and I started making my own products."

She began making bath oils, soaps, and lotions. "I learned how to blend essential oils into the products and I found them to be very useful for a number of things like clearing out blemishes, blotches, and break outs."

Around that time, she happened upon Nature's Sunshine, a health product distributorship. She took their aromatherapy classes and learned how to work with essential oils.

"Being a person of many feelings, I found a way to blend the essential oils depending on how I felt," Dean said. "When I was feeling sad, for example, I would use lavender oil to uplift me. I prefer blending just two or three oils together because the effect is better for me than if I blend more than three."

Dean makes soaps using glycerin base, which she sells among friends. "This is very mild soap that takes just 15 minutes to make," she said. "I add essential oils like tea tree, lavender, ylang-ylang, and peppermint and usually do not need to add color because the oils make their own color."

She also makes other products, including one that she calls "Sock it to me." It is a sock filled with crushed botanicals, other ingredients, and essential oils that can be warmed up in a microwave and used on sore parts of the body or placed on the nape of the neck to help the user inhale the essential oils.

"I suggest aromatherapy for everyone," Dean said. "It is safe, simple and in the long run, it is more economical than using store bought products. If you are just starting out, you should do your homework, find out what you like, and let everything you make be an expression of yourself."

Using products made from pure and natural ingredients can enhance the functions of your mind and body. The aromas from essential oils can stimulate the brain and heal the body and the following recipes can help.

Soaps

Once you graduate from the basic white soap recipe and you know how to add color, you have a wide range of different soaps that you can make. These include antiseptic soaps, floral soaps, fruit soaps, herbal soaps, spice soaps, and soaps made from other miscellaneous ingredients. Most soap makers name their soaps cleverly, depending on the kind of ingredients in each soap. Olive Splendor and Rosey Tosey are examples.

Antiseptic soap

Soap with antiseptic properties can help heal acne, cuts, insect bites, sunburns, and wounds. Make antiseptic soap at home with just a few natural ingredients.

INGREDIENTS

   3 cups glycerin base

   3 Tbsp. tea tree oil

   1 Tbsp. clove oil

DIRECTIONS

1.   Use the melt and pour method to prepare your ingredients.

2.   Pour your soap mixture in a mold, allow to firm up, and use.

Castile soap

Castile soap is probably the easiest and mildest soap to make at home. You can make it to use as a base for shampoos, bubble baths, and shower gels. Make it unscented and free of colorants for these uses.

INGREDIENTS

30 ounces olive oil

16 ounces water

10 ounces coconut oil

10 ounces palm oil

7 ounces lye

2 Tbsp. essential oil of choice (optional)

DIRECTIONS

1. Follow basic cold process soap making instructions by adding the lye to the water and dissolving it.

2. Mix your oils together.

3. Bring both mixtures to temperatures between 92 and 100 degrees and mix them together.

4. Bring to trace with a stick blender by stirring.

5. Store in a capped bottle.

Floral soap

You can make floral soap using the basic soap ingredients or the melt and pour method and later add floral essential oils, flower-infused oils, and floral additives like flower petals.

INGREDIENTS

3 cups clear or castile soap

1 cup distilled water

¼ cup lavender flowers

2 tsp. lavender oil

DIRECTIONS

1. Simmer lavender flowers in water for about five minutes then let steep overnight.

2. Strain resulting liquid.

3. Add into already melted glycerine soap base.

4. If you are making soap using either the cold process or hot process methods, use your infused lavender water in place of plain water.

5. Use color and mold shapes that match the flower ingredients in your soap for fun soaps.

Fruit soap

To make a fruity soap, you can use strawberries, peaches, mangos, and bananas in your soap mixture. Puree the fruits and add them to your oils.

Herbal soap

Herbal soap, like antiseptic soap, is good for helping heal the skin of common skin conditions like acne and eczema and helps keep a clear complexion. Use basic soap-making ingredients and the steps of either the cold or hot methods of soap making. Use herbal oils for fragrance and dried herbs for additives. You can also make an herbal infusion to use in your soap.

INGREDIENTS

16 ounces olive oil

8 ounces dried herbs like chamomile, patchouli, peppermint, and sage

DIRECTIONS

1. Combine the olive oil with your choice of herbs and let steep for at least 24 hours before using.

Shampoo

Good shampoo should clean your hair and not strip it of any natural oils. A basic shampoo recipe requires just a castile base, some water, fragrance, and additives.

Basic shampoo

INGREDIENTS

¼ cup castile soap

¾ cup distilled water

1 tsp. olive oil

2 drops essential oil of choice

DIRECTIONS

1. Mix all ingredients together and shake well before each use.

Bubble Bath

Making your own bubble bath can be fun, exciting, and economical. You can also add in the essential oil of your choice and practice aromatherapy while you relax in your bubble bath.

INGREDIENTS

4 cups liquid castile soap

4 cups distilled water

3 ounces glycerin, available at many health and vitamin stores

3 drops lavender or lemon oil

DIRECTIONS

1. Mix all ingredients together in a bowl.

2. Store in a squeeze bottle if available.

Use by pouring into running water for maximum bubble formation.

Shower Gel

Homemade shower gels are economical and allow you to customize them according to your scent preferences and needs.

INGREDIENTS

2 cups distilled water

8 Tbsp. aloe vera gel

4 Tbsp. glycerin

2 tsp. corn starch

2 tsp. jojoba oil

4 drops each of ylang-ylang, lavender, chamomile, and grapefruit oils

DIRECTIONS

1. Mix these ingredients well in a bowl.

2. Pour into any available squeeze bottle and use.

Store in the refrigerator to keep it fresh longer, or store in the bathroom cabinet and use within 30 days.

Laundry Soap

Instead of using potentially irritating, chemical-laden laundry detergents, make your laundry soap with just a few basic ingredients.

INGREDIENTS

12 cups water

1 cup washing soda, available in the laundry products aisle in the grocery store

1 cup Borax

20 drops lavender oil

1 homemade white bar soap

2-gallon bucket

DIRECTIONS

1. Grate the bar soap and mix with 6 cups of water before melting in a sauce pan.

2. Add the washing soda and Borax and stir until they dissolve.

3. Remove from heat and pour into the bucket.

4. Add the other 6 cups of water and essential oils and stir using a long handled plastic spoon until well mixed.

5. Use ½ a cup for each load of laundry. Leave the spoon in the bucket to stir the mixture before each use.

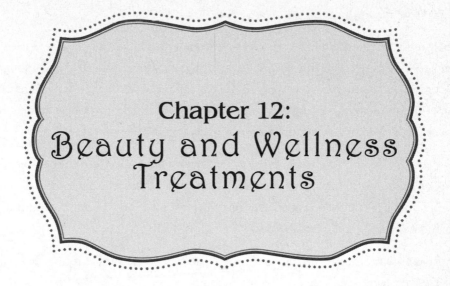

Chapter 12:
Beauty and Wellness Treatments

The beauty and wellness industry is full of choices. The only thing lacking from the industry is an assurance to consumers that using these products will not have short- or long-term negative side effects to their bodies. The only way to get this assurance is to take control of what goes into your body and know exactly how your body will react to the products you use.

Hands and Feet

Hands are said to give away a woman's true age and though women tend not to want to reveal their true ages, that should not be the only reason to take care of your hands. Similarly, wearing open toed and open back evening shoes should not be the only reason you exfoliate your feet. The beauty of aromatherapy is that you do not have to splurge on a manicure or a pedicure to get your hands and feet pampered and looking great. There are quick fixes and decadent, natural procedures that can help you achieve these goals.

• • •

Baths, soaks, and scrubs

Bathing your hands and feet requires an exfoliate like brown sugar blended with moisturizing jojoba oil and essential oils or an exfoliating, mild soap and enough warm water to cover the feet. Wet your hands and feet and then scrub them gently with the exfoliate, removing dead skin cells. This helps open up clogged pores so they can prepare to absorb any nourishing oils you use afterwards.

A good soak can be a tension reliever. Soak your hands and feet in the water for about five minutes then scrub them for another two minutes before rinsing them and applying hand and foot cream. You can do this once a week for beautifully exfoliated hands and feet.

You can make your own hand and foot scrub using this simple recipe that will leave your hands and feet soft and invigorated.

Lime and lavender scrub

INGREDIENTS

2 tsp. each lime and lavender essential oils

4 Tbsp. finely-ground apricot kernel shells

½ cup fresh or dried lavender flowers

¼ cup olive oil

DIRECTIONS

1. Use a blender to grind the apricot kernel shells and lavender flowers into very small bits.

2. Mix all your liquid ingredients in a small bowl then add your ground ingredients into the bowl of liquid ingredients, mixing well.

3. Use on your hands and feet by massaging into your hands and feet for up to five minutes. Rinse and repeat if necessary.

Minty eucalyptus powder

When you need more than a foot soak to get rid of sweaty feet, foot odor, or athlete's foot, fine foot powder made using essential oils and other ingredients can be irreplaceable. Foot powder made this way can also help relieve achy foot muscles.

INGREDIENTS

1 cup corn starch

5 drops peppermint, spearmint, and/or eucalyptus essential oils

DIRECTIONS

1. Use a blender to make your corn starch as fine as possible before adding the essential oils.

2. Mix well and package in empty spice shakers.

3. To use, shake the powder onto your feet.

Aloe vera and tea tree gel

Hand gels are used to kill germs and sanitize hands while you are on the go. You can easily make them at home.

INGREDIENTS

1 cup isopropyl alcohol

3 drops tea tree essential oil

1 cup aloe vera gel (available from natural body care retailers)

DIRECTIONS

1. Combine the alcohol with aloe vera gel in a plastic bottle.

2. Add essential oils, mix well, and use as needed.

Sweet almond and lavender cuticle oil

Cuticles ruining your near perfect manicure? Get rid of them easily by soaking and scrubbing your nails each week with a nail scrubber then use an orange stick, a small wooden stick with pointed ends that is available at most drug stores, to remove loose cuticle remnants. Later, you can apply cuticle oil to soften the cuticle area. Use the following recipe to make your own cuticle oil. Choose essential oils that have antiseptic properties as a way to protect your nails from fungus. Feel free to blend them with other fragrant essential oils that appeal to you.

INGREDIENTS

   2 teaspoons olive oil

   3 drops sweet almond essential oil

   1 drop lavender essential oil

DIRECTIONS

1. Combine all ingredients in a dark-colored glass bottle and mix well.
2. Massage into nails and cuticle areas. *Refer to Chapters 2 and 3 for proper storage requirements for carrier and essential oils.*

Butter foot balm

Hand and foot balm can help relieve soreness and also repair hands and feet that are dry, cracked, or otherwise damaged. Balm is a step above lotion because it is thicker and does not wash off easily, remaining on the skin longer for healing. Make your own balm by incorporating ingredients that you may already have in your home.

INGREDIENTS

   1 cup beeswax

   1 Tbsp. jojoba oil

   1 Tbsp. cocoa butter

   1 Tbsp. coconut oil

   ¼ cup shea butter

   15 to 20 drops essential oils like eucalyptus, peppermint, rosemary, and peppermint

DIRECTIONS

1. Melt your saturated oil ingredients using a double boiler on medium to low heat, taking care not to boil them.

2. Transfer the melted ingredients into a durable plastic container with a top.

3. Add one or a blend of essential oils, allow to cool, and use as necessary.

Minty foot lotion

Making your own foot lotion is useful when you want all natural ingredients going into your body just as aromatherapy calls for. This lotion is recommended for dry, callused skin and can be used to ease achy muscles.

INGREDIENTS

20 ounces melted beeswax from local beekeepers or online retailers

5 ounces essential oils, such as spearmint and peppermint

DIRECTIONS

1. Use a large metal or glass mixing bowl to combine the essential oils and the beeswax.

2. Mix well and transfer to a 24-ounce plastic container.

3. Massage onto your feet as necessary.

Paraffin wax mask

Masks for the hands and feet are often called paraffin treatments. They are a good way to lock in the moisture in the hands and feet so that they retain a soft and supple texture. Spas feature them on their menu boards, but they can also be easily made at home.

INGREDIENTS

4 ounces of paraffin wax, available from online retailers

2 to 4 drops olive oil

15 to 20 drops your choice of essential oil

Plastic wrap and/or plastic sandwich bags

DIRECTIONS

1. Use a double boiler to melt the paraffin.

2. Pour the paraffin into a mixing bowl and let it cool.

3. Smooth the olive oil onto your hands and feet.

4. Dip each foot and hand into the wax several times, creating several layers.

5. Wrap each hand and foot with the plastic wrap or place it into plastic sandwich bags.

6. Cover each hand and foot with a towel and wait 15 to 30 minutes to give the essential oils time to work. Peel off wax and discard.

Skin (Face and Body)

Skin care products like lotions can help you make the transformation, if you are not already there, toward healthiness. Try implementing one of the following recipes to create a new product you can incorporate into your beauty regiment.

Floral lotion

Just like with your hand and foot lotion, you can make lotion for your face and body inexpensively with exceptional moisturizing capabilities, fragrance, and all-natural ingredients. These ingredients should all go into a lotion base, which you can either make at home or buy ready made at a bath and body supply store.

INGREDIENTS

White, odorless lotion base

5 ounces fragrant blend of floral essential oils

2 to 4 drops color (optional)

DIRECTIONS

1. Pour the lotion base into a large metal or glass mixing bowl.

2. Mix your coloring and essential oils into the lotion base using a spatula.

3. Use a funnel to transfer the resulting mixture into plastic bottles with airtight tops.

4. Use this lotion on your hands, feet, and skin as necessary and store in a cool place away from light.

Masks

If you like to experiment, you know that you can make face masks out of some of the food you have in your home. These face masks are a great way to have a spa day at home while removing the impurities harboring in your pores.

Clay mask for oily skin

INGREDIENTS

1 ounce bentonite clay from online or local mineral retailers (this clay will draw out impurities in the skin)

2 Tbsp. water

1 Tbsp. carrot oil

1 egg yolk

1 drop grapefruit oil

DIRECTIONS

1. Mix the clay with all the other ingredients and apply it on the face and throat.

2. Let the mixture sit for ten to 15 minutes, then wash off with warm water.

Aloe vera mask for dry and sensitive skin

INGREDIENTS

3 Tbsp. aloe vera juice (you can purchase this at health food stores)

1 Tbsp. aloe vera gel

3 drops essential oils of your choice

DIRECTIONS

1. Mix all the ingredients up in a bowl and stir well.

2. Use cotton balls to apply it on your face and neck.

3. Leave the mask on for up to ten minutes then rinse off with warm water.

Facial steams

You should use a steam once or twice a week for clean, unclogged pores. Steams are probably the simplest way to have a spa treatment at home. All you will need to do is sit at a table with your face over a hot bowl of water enhanced with some essential oils and a towel over your head.

INGREDIENTS

½ gallon clean water in a kettle

2 drops minty or herby essential oils like peppermint or tea tree oil

½ cup fresh or dried herbs (optional)

DIRECTIONS

1. Boil the water and transfer it into a large bowl.

2. Add essential oils or herbs to the hot water.

3. Place a towel over your head and place your face over the large bowl, allowing the steam from the bowl to purify your face.

Cleansers and toners

The combination of cleansers and toners works well because cleansers were traditionally oily and toners made with alcohol could get rid of the oily residue they left behind. Today, cleansers are rarely oily but toners, which no longer contain alcohol, can have toning effects on the skin.

Oatmeal cleanser

INGREDIENTS

½ cup oatmeal, ground to a fine dust

2 Tbsp. heavy cream

DIRECTIONS

1. Mix both ingredients well and apply on face with strokes moving away from your face.

2. Let the mixture sit for ten minutes, then rinse well using warm water.

Chamomile and honey toner

INGREDIENTS

½ cup distilled water

½ tsp. chamomile essential oil

2 tsp. honey

2 tsp. vegetable oil

DIRECTIONS

1. Mix the ingredients well and apply on your face.

2. Let it work for ten minutes before rinsing with warm water.

Shea butter and jojoba balm

Body balms can be especially useful during the winter moths when cold air drains your skin of moisture. This simple body balm recipe will help your skin and face prepare for winter without dread.

INGREDIENTS

2 ounces shea butter

2 ounces jojoba oil

1 ounce cocoa butter

½ ounce beeswax

10 drops floral essential oil

10 drops orange essential oil

5 drops rosemary essential oil

DIRECTIONS

1. Place the beeswax, cocoa butter, and shea butter in a double boiler to slowly melt.

2. Mix in all the other ingredients and stir well.

3. Allow to cool slightly before transferring into a sterilized plastic container with a lid.

Sesame serum

Serums can be used on the face and body to protect the skin against sun damage. The skin will absorb them quickly and when they are made using certain oils, like sesame oil and jojoba, they moisturize and stimulate collagen creation.

INGREDIENTS

3 Tbsp. sesame oil

3 Tbsp. jojoba oil

5 drops carrot oil

5 drops Roman chamomile oil

DIRECTIONS

1. Melt the jojoba and mix ingredients in a small dropper bottle.
2. Apply to clean face with special attention to avoid the eye areas.

Lips

Lips require tender loving care because they are prone to falling victims to conditions — wind, cold, sunlight — that can cause them to crack. This can not only make for a very painful condition, but it can also leave them susceptible to infections such as herpes. The best way to protect them is to coat them with lip balms.

Almond and jojoba balm

The days of solely petroleum-based lips balms are gone. You can now make balms with alternative and natural ingredients that are nourishing and soothing. As with many of the beauty and wellness products already featured, balms can incorporate base and essential oils.

INGREDIENTS

1 Tbsp. melted beeswax

½ Tbsp. sweet almond oil

10 drops jojoba oil

10 drops chamomile essential oil

1 capsule of vitamin E

DIRECTIONS

1. Stir the beeswax and almond oil together.

2. Add jojoba, the vitamin E, and the chamomile oil.

3. Pour into a small, easy to carry plastic container with a lid. Use this balm after it firms up, either at room temperature or in a refrigerator.

Teeth and Gums

Bright white, healthy teeth are not always the product of dentists or commercially available toothpaste, toothbrushes, and mouthwash. Traditionalist Africans have used aromatherapy for dental health and hygiene for centuries and they have bright smiles and strong teeth. Research has shown that the sticks these Africans chew on contain antibiotics, fluoride, and other anti-cavity ingredients. In fact the World Health Organization (WHO) promotes chewing on twigs from the *salvadora persica* tree as a natural toothbrush.

This story from the other side of the world should serve as inspiration that nature, indeed, has a way of taking care of you. And even though you might be apprehensive about giving up what you are used to, you can never know the benefits of the alternative until you try it.

Peppermint mouthwash

You can save a few dollars every few weeks by giving the baking soda in your refrigerator another chore. Baking soda serves as the lead ingredient in your homemade mouthwash and it protects and freshens your mouth just as well as — if not better than — the store-bought varieties.

INGREDIENTS

2 ounces water

¼ tsp. baking soda

1 drop peppermint oil

1 drop tea tree oil

DIRECTIONS

Mix all the ingredients in a plastic bottle and shake well before use.

Clove teeth powder

Teeth cleaning powders should not only give the user fresh breath, they should also kill bacteria in the mouth and promote teeth whitening. If you have teeth fillers or artificial teeth and other teeth products, research the effect of certain essential oils on them. Oregano oil, for example, can stain bonding.

INGREDIENTS

3 tsp. baking soda

1 tsp. table or sea salt

1 drop clove oil

DIRECTIONS

Mix well in a small container and use with your toothbrush every day in place of toothpaste.

Hair

The market for hair products is vast, which is evident in the $60 billion United States consumers spend on beauty products each year. Here are some hair care recipes you can follow using some of your favorite essential oils.

Rinses

A good hair rinse should leave your hair and scalp clean and shiny without using additives and chemicals like sodium lauryl sulfate that can irritate the scalp or other chemicals that are harmful. Using natural ingredients can save you money while protecting your hair, scalp, and body.

Honey lemon rinse

4 cups warm water

3 Tbsp. lemon juice

2 tsp. honey

DIRECTIONS

1. Massage the rinse of your choice over your freshly-washed hair and wash off after five minutes.

2. Note that the natural acidity in the lemon juice may give you blond highlights with frequent use.

Herbal sage rinse

INGREDIENTS

1 cup hot water

1 Tbsp. dried sage

DIRECTIONS

1. Place the sage in a heat resistant bowl and pour water over it.

2. Let it steep until it cools down to a comfortable temperature.

3. Strain and use on freshly-washed hair, massaging it gently for up to five minutes.

Oils

We all need to oil our hair to help boost shine and get rid of dry scalp. Using aromatherapy oils has several benefits beyond the obvious for hair and scalp. A blend of the right essential oils can promote hair growth and prevent dandruff as well. For oily hair, a blend of basil and rosemary oils can work well for both issues. For dry hair, a blend of carrot oil mixed with jojoba oil can help stimulate underactive sebaceous glands, promoting natural oil to counter dry scalp. Adding geranium oil to either blend group can help strengthen hair.

All-around hair blend

INGREDIENTS

3 drops basil oil

3 drops rosemary oil

3 drops carrot oil

3 drops lavender oil

4 ounces jojoba oil

DIRECTIONS

Mix all oils well in a plastic container and massage into scalp at least twice a week.

Aloe vera hair gel

Gels can be used to make the hair look thicker and more voluminous. They also make hair easier to style and help you maintain the hairstyles you work so hard to achieve while controlling any natural frizz you might have.

INGREDIENTS

1 cup aloe vera gel

1 cup warm water

½ tsp. unflavored gelatin

½ tsp. rose (or preferred) oil

DIRECTIONS

1. In a plastic or other container with a lid, add the aloe vera gel and gelatin to the warm water.

2. Add the rose essential oil and mix all the ingredients together until the mixture is smooth and thick.

3. If it is too watery, add a bit more gelatin and if it is too thick, add a bit more water.

4. Use as necessary and store in the refrigerator when not in use. This recipe works well on any type of hair texture, ethnic or otherwise.

Detangling serums

Combing hair can be torturous when it is tangled. Mothers of young daughters, especially, know just how much. Detangling hair is a necessary ritual to not only avoid dreadlocks but to also avoid chemicals and preservatives.

INGREDIENTS

4 ounces distilled water

15 drops grapefruit oil

3 drops glycerin

3 drops orange oil

1 tsp. aloe vera gel

Bottle

DIRECTIONS

Mix all your ingredients in the bottle and use as needed.

Dry shampoo

Dry clean your hair to remove extra oil or when you are in a rush to get ready. Dry cleaning is also very useful for bed-stricken individuals and the elderly.

INGREDIENTS

½ cup cornstarch

2 drops basil or rosemary oil

DIRECTIONS

1. Mix the two ingredients well.

2. Slowly add some of the mixture into your hair.

3. Let the dry shampoo sit on your head for up to ten minutes before brushing it out. Keep in mind that cornstarch can be messy, so use it sparingly.

Conditioners

Use some of these recipes to nourish and soften hair after shampooing. Using a good conditioner can protect your hair from getting dreaded split ends while adding luster and shine to the hair.

Egg and avocado conditioner

INGREDIENTS

- 1 cup avocado, seedless and skinless
- 2 egg yolks
- 1 Tbsp. rosemary oil

DIRECTIONS

1. Mix the ingredients in a blender until smooth.
2. Apply to your hair and leave in for 30 minutes.
3. Rinse with warm water and repeat after each shampoo.

Rosemary conditioner

INGREDIENTS

- 5 drops rosemary oil
- 1 Tbsp. jojoba oil

DIRECTIONS

1. Blend well and massage into hair.
2. Wrap with a towel and leave in for up to an hour.
3. Unwrap and style without rinsing.

Coconut deodorant

Using deodorants is a very important grooming ritual meant to prevent and mask odor caused by perspiration. Commercially available deodorants are alcohol-based with chemical additives like aluminium chlorohydrate to kill these bacteria, but homemade deodorants can work just as well with less harsh ingredients.

INGREDIENTS

¼ cup baking soda

¼ cup cornstarch

5 Tbsp. spruce or sandalwood oil

DIRECTIONS

1. Combine the baking soda and cornstarch then add your essential oil.

2. Place the mixture in a sanitized container with a lid.

3. Mix well until it reaches a desirable consistency that you can either scoop into your old deodorant dispenser or leave in the container to apply with your clean fingers with each use.

Massage Oils

Considered a small luxury for many Americans, a good massage can do wonders for the body. Different massage techniques and different massage oils exist to complement the part of the body being massaged and the reason for the massage. For example, Swedish massage is very gentle and relaxing, which is good for easing tension, while deep tissue massage is good for chronically tight and painful muscles or repetitive strain. Additionally, lavender oil is good for calming so when the occasion calls for a soothing blend, why not use it?

Massage oil blends

You can create massage oils to complement different moods in your life or what you want to accomplish. Oils can be blended to be sensual, soothing, and stimulating. You can also blend them to complement similar fragrances.

Sensual blend

If you are looking to ignite that loving feeling, blend massage oils including clary sage, jasmine, patchouli, rose, sandalwood, or ylang-ylang.

INGREDIENTS

10 drops sandalwood oil

5 drops rose oil

5 drops bergamot oil

1.5 ounces sweet almond or grapeseed oil

DIRECTIONS

Mix all your ingredients together in a dark-colored container of an appropriate size and use as needed.

Soothing blend

Life's many problems got you feeling a little blue and needing some uplifting? How about a quick ten-minute soothing massage? Use the blend below for a quick fix.

INGREDIENTS

15 drops neroli oil

3 drops black pepper oil

2 drops rosemary oil

1.5 ounces grapeseed oil

DIRECTIONS

Mix well and use as necessary. Inhaling this blend can also offer uplifting benefits to the user.

Stimulating blend

A stimulating massage oil blend can help increase blood circulation to the muscles and relieve muscle soreness.

INGREDIENTS

10 drops geranium oil

5 drops cypress oil

5 drops thyme oil

1.5 ounces jojoba oil

DIRECTIONS

Mix well and use as needed.

Floral blend

Try the following combination to create a nice floral blend that fills the nostrils with the soft aroma of flowers.

INGREDIENTS

10 drops lavender oil

8 drops jasmine oil

2 drops rose oil

DIRECTIONS

Mix well and use as necessary.

CASE STUDY: LAURIE D. ANDREWS

The Natural Therapy Center
2520-D Professional Rd.
Richmond, Va. 23235
804-267-3477 Office
804-916-9494 Cell
laurie@thenaturaltherapycenter.com
www.thenaturaltherapycenter.com

Laurie Andrews started the Natural Therapy Center to teach others how to "heal the body, mind, and spirit through natural remedies, hands-on body work, and knowledge." She teaches classes to help the public learn about aromatherapy and help them understand that "our bodies are of the earth, not chemical made. This is why we react to chemical products, which give us negative side effects, but we thrive when we use natural products."

Andrews studied natural health for several years before embarking on entrepreneurship. In the late 1990s, she studied advanced clinical massage and bodywork therapies at the Utah College of Massage Therapy as well as taking courses in relaxation therapy and natural health consulting.

In 1999, Andrews began teaching in massage and bodywork schools, rising to director of the new massage therapy department at Tidewater Tech in Hampton Roads, Va., before opening her own school for massage therapy in 2006. She is licensed as a massage therapist in Utah and is a certified massage therapist in Virginia and has published numerous articles on her craft.

Andrews now wears many hats — as a natural health consultant, relaxation therapist, aromatherapy instructor, and Reiki master, among others. As a Reiki master, she practices Reiki, a Japanese technique of healing used for promoting relaxation and reducing stress. It is based on laying hands and the belief that unseen energy flows from one person to another.

She teaches aromatherapy to new users by helping them understand essential oil basics and how they work in basic biology, such as how the olfactory system's relationship with the brain can promote healing to the rest of the body when a user inhales essential oils. "The benefits reach the body faster this way. I use this mode frequently and I have not been sick for years," Andrews said.

Andrews recommends that everyone have the essential oil of lavender with them at all times. "It has so many positives — it is relaxing, it can help with insomnia, bruising, headaches. It is a great antiviral and antibacterial. I take it with me when I stay at hotels, which really creep me out, and use a few drops on the bed sheets and pillows to kill bed mites and make the place smell great."

Perfumes

A plethora of perfumes exist in the market. They can be overwhelming, heady, and worse, not unique. This happens even despite the fact that commercial perfumes can contain more than 250 ingredients per bottle. Blending essential oils, on the contrary, requires just a few good smelling ingredients that include distilled water, essential oils, and 100-proof vodka to accentuate the aroma of the essential oils and offer antibacterial properties. If you are making perfumed oil, you can add carrier oil like jojoba into the mix.

The perfume you like should make you want to inhale its scent on your wrist several times a day while causing you to wonder if others around you enjoy it too. Finding what you like is unique and what you like should be fun and exciting.

How to choose your favorite scent

Perfume scents are divided into the same aromatic blends covered in Chapter 6. Citrus scents can energize you; earthy scents can be mysterious; and floral scents can make you relax and smile. Additionally, herbal, minty, spicy, and woody scents can be warming, grounding, and energizing. Whatever scents you find appealing are the scents you should use for your perfume.

Supplies and equipment

To make your own perfume from essential oils, you will need to have the following items:

- Droppers

- Funnel

- Measuring cups

- Measuring spoons

- Glass rod

- Electric coffee mill (available where appliances are sold) to dry flowers if your recipe calls for it

Blending

Blending perfume scents is similar to blending essential oil scents. Consider the fragrance notes covered in Chapter 6 and start out small by blending just two or three scents at first. Any more than three can become overpowering and prevent you from enjoying your perfume.

Bottling and storage

Your local craft store is a good place to find all the bottles and storage supplies you need for your perfumes. Purchase dark bottles to store your creations and, because they contain volatile essential oils, store them in a cool, dark place away from heat and light. The bathroom is not the best place to store them.

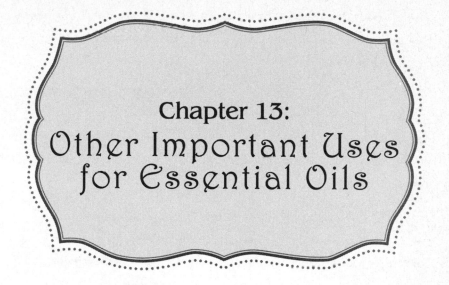

Chapter 13:
Other Important Uses for Essential Oils

Every daily activity can be potentially touched by essential oils. And by extension, the lives of pets can be touched as well. In this chapter, learn how you can uses essential oils for pets and for other loved ones, whether at homes or in other facilities.

Pets

Alternative care for your furry friends, large and small, is neither a strange nor a new idea. Often times people treat their pets like beloved family members so knowing that they can benefit from aromatherapy just as much as humans do is reason enough to pursue such care. Essential oils can help ease the aches and pains pets develop from play, disease, and old age, while getting rid of fleas, ticks, and foul odors.

Pet aromatherapy professionals recommend using diffusion to get essential oils into your pets. This involves using a diffuser to release or diffuse essential oils into the air in an enclosed space. This can be in a house, kennel, barn, or any place where you can find animals and is considered very safe. The diffused oils are then inhaled and as they travel from the nose or mouth through the rest of

• • •

an animal's body, they impart their fragrance and trigger numerous beneficial stimulations. Essential oils can also be administered by using them in pet products such as shampoos.

Safety points to consider

Always dilute essentials oils with carrier oils before using them on small pets. In larger animals such as horses, essential oils can be used neat. Use just enough to rub into the animal's coat.

Some pet aromatherapy professionals do not recommend using essential oils for birds or cats but others do. The best rule to subscribe to when you are unsure is to consult with a qualified health practitioner, in this case, a veterinarian.

Calming lavender blend

Emotional issues such as fear, anxiety, stress, and confusion can affect animal temperament and cause your pet to act out, become loud, or ignore directions and lessons. Lavender and citrus essential oils, both of which have calming properties, are favorites to help dissipate these emotional issues.

INGREDIENTS

20 drops lavender oil

10 drops chamomile oil

10 drops rose geranium

DIRECTIONS

Blend well in a clean, small glass container, add to a diffuser, and enjoy.

Flea and tick blend

Fleas and ticks are probably the cause of many pet owners' distress but they can be easily remedied without using chemical-based detergents that pose possibly adverse side effects like skin irritation, sores, hair loss, vomiting, and even damaged organs. Always consult a veterinarian for more serious flea and tick infestations.

INGREDIENTS

3 cups distilled water

2 drops basil

2 drops cedarwood

1 tsp. vodka for extra antiseptic

DIRECTIONS

Blend all ingredients in a spray bottle and spray on your pet's coat.

Cleaning and freshening blend

Pet odors do not have to be in control of your home. Use the following recipe to fight bad pet odor even on a damp, rainy day.

INGREDIENTS

8 ounces water

10 drops lavender

3 drops Roman chamomile

3 drops geranium

3 drops sweet marjoram

DIRECTIONS

Mix well in a spray bottle and spray on your pet's coat while avoiding the face and eyes.

Pet soap

This recipe will produce a gentle soap that can repel fleas and ticks while deodorizing your pet's fur.

INGREDIENTS

½ pound glycerin soap base

5 drops citronella oil

5 drops lavender oil

1 tsp. jojoba oil

1 tsp. shea butter

1 tsp. beeswax

DIRECTIONS

1. Use a double boiler to melt your ingredients.

2. Add essential oils and mix well.

3. Pour into molds and bang on counter to remove air bubbles.

4. Let firm up either in a freezer for 30 minutes to an hour, or at room temperature for several hours and use as necessary.

Elderly Loved Ones

The elderly have weakened immune systems and are more susceptible to infections. Contemporary medicine recommends using vitamins and shots to counter these lurking dangers, but aromatherapy is a viable alternative to conventional medicine and offers many benefits. The benefits from using essential oil blends include naturally boosting immune systems to keep away infections and increase mental acuity.

Choosing the best essential oils for the individuals

Remember that the elderly have thinner skin, which can be more prone to irritation from improperly diluted essential oils. Beyond that, choose essential oils that can give them the most benefit, depending on the condition that is afflicting the intended individual. Choose lemongrass because of its aroma and ability to ease stress and relieve muscle soreness. Choose peppermint because of its refreshing properties, ability to stimulate the senses, and ability to treat minor ailments.

In hospitals and nursing homes

Despite their functions as healing centers, hospitals can be inadvertent germ-exchange centers. People with communicable diseases such as tuberculosis can pass along their germs to the healthy and increase cross infections. Realizing this, some hospitals such as Memorial Sloan-Kettering Cancer Center in New York have began to use aromatherapy and especially essential oils, to help increase patient and visitor well being. Much like hospitals, nursing homes are strongholds for germs and germ-swapping. Using a diffuser in the room of a loved one can protect him or her from some of these germs.

Traveling

Those long lines at airport security checkpoints can be frustrating but probably not as irritating as catching an infection from a fellow traveler. When you are travelling, pack essential oils in your bags so you can use them as necessary.

Packing essential oils such as lavender and cedarwood can help you easily deal with the stress of travel, including motion sickness. You can carry them to help ease minor discomforts — a spritzer when it is hot and some peppermint oil on a cotton ball or handkerchief can help ease headaches. An aromatherapy trip kit with oils such as lavender tea tree should not contain liquids in more than 3 ounce bottles to comply with Transportation Security Administration (TSA) standards.

Workplace

Using scent in the workplace can make it a more appealing place to be. If you are the boss, using scents may be a way to increase employee productivity without uttering a word. And if you are the employee, you might find yourself enjoying the atmosphere so much that an eight-hour shift feels more like a four-hour shift. This all depends on the oils you choose to use in diffusers and aroma lamps that can be strategically placed in the workplace.

Gender-neutral oils will work best in a workplace. Citrus oils like lemon and spicy oils like clary sage are good starting points. Also choose oils that can treat workplace stress. Bergamot has antidepressant and sedative effects, while lemon will clear the mind and grapefruit can be uplifting.

Pregnancy and Childbirth

Although seeking qualified medical advice is recommended before using essential oils during pregnancy, several essential oils are considered safe to use when diluted well, according to the National Association for Holistic Aromatherapy (NAHA). These essential oils include: chamomile, geranium, jasmine, lavender, neroli, patchouli, sandalwood, and ylang-ylang. These oils can be very helpful in easing the pains and discomforts that come along with pregnancy, childbirth, and baby care.

Morning sickness is an early discomfort of pregnancy for many women but if you are lucky enough to avoid it in the first few months of pregnancy, there will likely be other pains and discomforts you will experience during pregnancy. While your rapidly stretching belly itches and threatens to invite in ugly stretch marks, the extra weight you are carrying will begin to make your back ache. The extra fluids in your body also will likely make your legs swell.

For centuries, pregnant women have courageously suffered these consequences, but with the following aromatherapy recipes, women can gain beautiful families without experiencing the worst of these discomforts.

Backache fighting blend

INGREDIENTS

8 drops cinnamon oil

6 drops Roman chamomile oil

4 drops ginger oil

1 Tbsp. almond oil

DIRECTIONS

Mix all the oils and use as massage oil on the back.

Soothing swollen legs

Fluid retention during pregnancy is a common problem usually in the third trimester. This problem, called edema or dropsy, is more visible on the legs and feet. You will need highly a concentrated essential oil blend for a foot soak to help with this problem.

INGREDIENTS

1 ounce pumpkin seed oil

20 drops cypress oil

20 drops fennel oil

DIRECTIONS

Combine all of the ingredients and soak your feet for 20 minutes.

Soothing massage for calmness

Calmness does not often go hand in hand with labor and delivery, especially if the childbirth is all natural. Incorporating aromatherapy into this process can be useful for mothers who choose to go the completely natural route, whether in a hospital with doctors or at home with a midwife.

INGREDIENTS

4 drops eucalyptus, lavender, or peppermint oil

3 ounces almond oil

DIRECTIONS

Use this simple blend to massage the back, neck, and other parts of the body as needed.

Cocoa butter and beeswax cream

Cocoa butter is the highly praised stretch mark balm and for good reason. It helps keep the skin soft and can prevent stretch marks from developing or diminish the appearance of existing stretch marks. Cocoa butter exists in many costly brand names, but you can glean its many benefits by making your own inexpensive blend.

INGREDIENTS

½ cup cocoa butter

1 Tbsp. apricot kernel oil

1 Tbsp. wheat germ oil

2 tsp. grated beeswax

5 drops cedarwood oil

5 drops rosemary oil

DIRECTIONS

1. Melt the beeswax and mix with other ingredients. Apply by massaging to affected areas twice or three times a day.

Olive oil stretch mark cream

Other home remedies involve using olive oil and aloe vera, known for soothing and healing burns. The following recipe calls for aloe vera to prevent and treat stretch marks.

INGREDIENTS

½ cup olive oil

¼ cup aloe vera gel

DIRECTIONS

Blend ingredients together and store in an airtight container in the refrigerator.

Baby Care

Practicing aromatherapy before and during pregnancy will make extending the practice into your baby's care easier. Being health conscious gives your baby a very good chance at fighting and beating common ailments found in infants and children. When using essential oils on babies, make sure you dilute them more than you would if using them on an adult.

Baths and oils

You can give your baby a gentle aromatic bath by adding one to three drops of lavender essential oil and Roman chamomile essential oil to the baby's bath water.

Diaper changes

Aromatherapy offers simple ways to prevent and treat diaper rash in conjunction with frequent diaper changes. The following is a basic recipe you can use on your infant.

INGREDIENTS

2 Tbsp. castor oil

2 Tbsp. olive oil

1½ tsp. beeswax

½ tsp. vitamin E oil

10 drops lavender or tea tree oil

DIRECTIONS

1. Melt the beeswax and mix with the other oils for use as necessary.

2. You can let the blend stay on the skin without rinsing it off.

3. Store in a cool place in a container with a lid.

Using Aromatherapy in Schools

Imagine a world where everyone uses aromatherapy. It would be a calmer, more friendly world as aroma works its way into our minds and imparts its healing on every walk of life. Schools can also benefit from aromatherapy much like employees in the workplace. Relaxed minds, and decluttered minds, can lead to better learning skills and increased memory and concentration. Parents can easily send essential oils to school by adding a few drops of oils such as hyssop, lemon, or tea tree on cotton balls or a handkerchief and placing them in a plastic sandwich bag. Your student can then inhale the aroma every time he or she is feeling distracted or overwhelmed. Teachers and educators can also use essential oils in their classrooms and offices, perhaps in a diffuser.

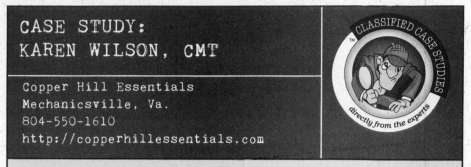

CASE STUDY:
KAREN WILSON, CMT

Copper Hill Essentials
Mechanicsville, Va.
804-550-1610
http://copperhillessentials.com

Karen Wilson suggests that using essential oils and aromatherapy in general should start out slowly so that people learn all they can. To achieve that, she loves to give tips on how to properly use essential oils to combat minor illnesses — using french lavender for cuts and scrapes, eucalyptus for colds, and lemon and tea tree as antiseptics.

Wilson, proprietor of Copper Hill Essentials, sells her aromatic and therapeutic wares through her website and at local natural food stores in central Virginia. She also sells them to area hospitals, which have began to understand the benefits of aromatherapy products and use peppermint drops in the toilet to help women who have just given birth have easier bowel movements. Through these venues, Wilson continually shares the knowledge she has gained in the last 20-plus years to those interested. "The natural scents are storehouses of energies, which can bring love, prosperity, happiness, psychic awareness, peace, and protection," she said.

Wilson believes every family can incorporate aromatherapy and essential oils into their lives and reap the myriad benefits they offer. "They are all natural, have fewer side effects, promote physical and emotional well-being. Who would not want to be a part of that?"

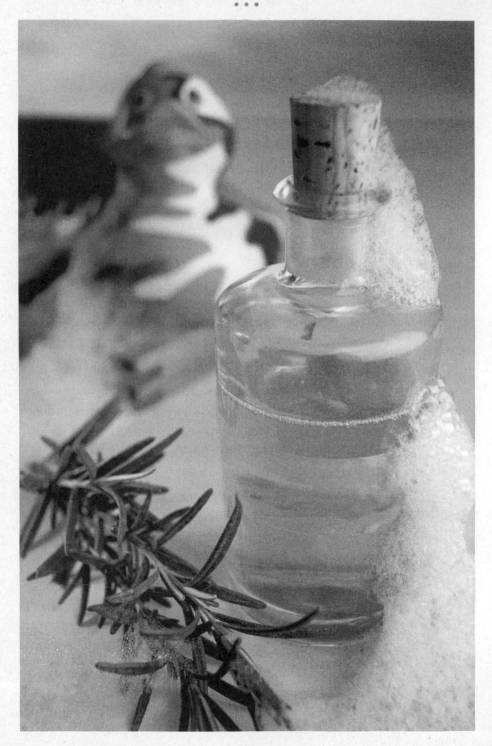

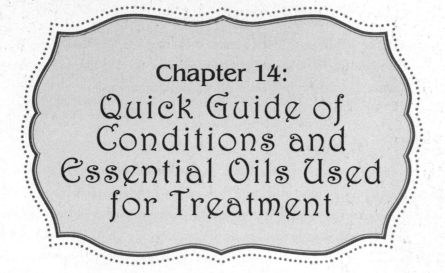

Chapter 14:
Quick Guide of Conditions and Essential Oils Used for Treatment

Simple essential oil treatments exist for minor conditions. These treatments are both rich in aroma and useful in therapy, just as aromatherapy calls for, and they can be administered in many different ways, including in massage therapy, vapor therapy, bath oils, and even in food. Common sense and top-notch judgment are important when using essential oils, because they are very powerful agents that can injure a user who does not follow precautions.

Precautions

Always use essential oils in a dilution, especially if children, the frail, and/or the elderly will use them. Always seek professional medical advice when in doubt about the condition you are seeking to alleviate. For conditions such as diabetes, kidney disease, and cancer, you should not rely on essential oils although they can help.

Physical Conditions

Any conditions afflicting the outer body, including the skin, are included in this description. The following recipes will help you prepare simple homemade treatments for some of the most common physical conditions.

Acne

Acne is hardly just a teenage problem. It also affects adults and can be very upsetting, because it robs people of their self-esteem and confidence. Today, numerous topical and electrolysis treatments, like lasers, exist. Other treatments like topical gels may sometimes clear up the acne but do nothing to take care of the deep-rooted conditions like overactive oil glands and clogged pores that cause flare-ups. Essential oils, on the other hand, are simple, non-invasive treatments that can work on both the external acne and the internal triggers that cause it.

INGREDIENTS

6 drops tea tree oil

5 drops rosewood oil

5 drops geranium oil

5 drops lavender oil

1 ounce distilled water

DIRECTIONS

1. Use a cotton ball to dab the blend on the affected areas for several days until they are clear.

2. You can also make this blend a part of a weekly facial regimen by cleaning the face, using steams or a mask, and then dabbing the blend all over the face. You do not have to wash off this diluted blend unless its aroma bothers you.

Addiction blend

Alcohol, cigarettes, drugs — legal and illegal — are the most common causes of addiction in the United States. Addiction develops for many reasons, but most often occur when people are unable to balance their personal issues with their emotions. Using alcohol, cigarettes, and drugs often masks these emotions or dulls the intensity of these emotions.

Programs like Alcoholics Anonymous in conjunction with rehabilitation can usually help addicts confront their feelings and help them work toward ending their addictions. Aromatherapy can also help calm the emotions like anxiety and stress that drive people to seek destructive behaviors. Inhaling essential oils each time the urge to use these intoxicants comes on triggers the brain's limbic region, which controls emotions and actions. In time — about three months — the strength of the essential oils in the blend can diminish the urge to smoke.

INGREDIENTS

10 drops jasmine oil

5 drops bergamot oil

5 drops sandalwood oil

DIRECTIONS

1. Blend well and use in a burner or vaporizers or dilute in 1 ounce jojoba oil to use on skin.

2. A drop or two on the back of the hand is sufficient for inhalation.

Allergies blend

When you feel a sore throat coming on or you have a sinus headache from allergies, use a blend of diluted essential oils to combat your allergy symptoms.

INGREDIENTS

10 drops clove oil

10 drops lemon oil

5 drops cinnamon bark oil

5 drops eucalyptus oil

5 drops rosemary oil

2 ounces sweet almond oil

DIRECTIONS

1. Mix well in a dark-colored dropper bottle and use up to eight drops internally in your food or drink and externally by direct inhalation.

2. For direct inhalation, put a drop of the diluted essential oil blend on the back of your hand and inhale it for several minutes.

Arthritis and rheumatism blend

This common condition afflicts mostly the elderly, inflames joints, and causes severe pain. Anti-inflammatory essential oils like Roman chamomile and black pepper do not cure arthritis but when used in conjunction with a healthy diet and exercise, they can significantly minimize flare-ups.

INGREDIENTS

10 drops Roman chamomile

3 drops black pepper

1 ounce jojoba oil

DIRECTIONS

1. Blend the oils well in a dark-colored bottle.

2. Use a drop at a time to massage into aching joints.

3. Seek medical advice on methods of massage, because different types of arthritis may call for different methods of massage.

Asthma blend

A sometimes severe respiratory condition, asthma is characterized by recurrent attacks and is often managed by inhalers that contain pharmaceutical medications that can have negative side effects like dry mouth, ear pain, headaches, increased heart rate, insomnia, and throat irritation. Essential oils with calming and decongestant qualities such as cedarwood, eucalyptus, frankincense, geranium, and pine work well to treat asthma.

INGREDIENTS

20 drops hazelnut oil

8 drops lavender oil

2 drops Roman chamomile oil

DIRECTIONS

1. Once the blend has been mixed well, massage a few drops on the chest in between asthma attacks and at bedtime.

2. The blend can also be used in bath water or in a steam treatment.

Athlete's foot blend

Three different types of fungus that all favor warm, moist areas between the toes cause this common fungal infection. The infection can also affect nails, groin area, scalp, and beard and is characterized by scaling, itchiness, blisters, and rashes. Over the counter and prescription treatments exist, but they are often chemical-laden and can have negative side effects. Using essential oils in conjunction with keeping feet dry and out of tight shoes can eradicate the infection.

INGREDIENTS

8 drops tea tree oil

4 drops peppermint oil

2 drops lavender oil

DIRECTIONS

1. Dilute at 50 percent with a base oil of choice and apply directly on the feet, making sure the blend covers every affected part of the foot. There is no need to wash off these good oils.

Backache blend

Backaches affect millions of Americans every year as a result of occupational or general injury, childbirth, poor posture, obesity, stress, and infection. It is the second most common reason for visits to the doctor, second only to upper respiratory ailments. The American Chiropractic Association, a professional association representing chiropractic doctors, recommends treating backaches by spinal manipulation, which involves many twists and turns. An alternative treatment lies in the use of essential oils to relax back muscles and provide relief for minor and some severe aches.

INGREDIENTS

15 drops lavender oil

10 drops rosemary oil

5 drops lemon oil

1 ounce almond oil

DIRECTIONS

Blend the oils together in a dark-colored bottle and use to massage affected area daily or as needed.

Bronchitis blend

This upper respiratory infection very often succeeds colds. It is characterized by coughs and congestion, which can be painful to watch and listen to, especially in young children. Thankfully camphoric essential oils can quickly help dissipate these symptoms.

INGREDIENTS

8 drops peppermint oil

7 drops lemon oil

5 drops sage oil

5 drops clove oil

DIRECTIONS

This blend can be massaged on the chest or used in a diffuser, allowing the camphor in the oils to treat inflammation and congestion in the chest.

No more bruises blend

Bruises often turn an ugly purplish, black, and blue color after just a few hours but did you know this could be minimized and even avoided if you administer aromatherapy first aid as soon as an area is injured? Spicy and resinous oils are particularly useful for this type of treatment, because they draw warmth to the injured area, increasing blood flow and allowing the skin to reabsorb and disperse the blood trapped in the bruised area.

INGREDIENTS

6 drops clove oil

4 drops black pepper oil

3 drops peppermint oil

2 drops marjoram oil

2 drops geranium oil

2 drops cypress oil

DIRECTIONS

Once the blend has been well mixed in a glass bottle, apply to each affected area by massaging gently at least twice a day.

Soothing burn blend

Whether the burn is from the sun or another heat source, it is bound to be painful and slow healing. Aromatherapists love to use oils that reduce the burning sensation and hasten cell regeneration. These oils include chamomile, geranium, lavender, peppermint, and tea tree oil.

INGREDIENTS

- 15 drops aloe vera
- 5 drops lavender oil
- 5 drops Roman chamomile oil

DIRECTIONS

Mix well and apply gently on the burned surface.

Candida

Quite simply, this is a yeast infection usually found in moist areas like the mucus membranes in the mouth, intestinal tract, and vagina where it is the cause of a painful itch. By the time symptoms become evident, the good bacteria in the body that usually feasts on candida have been overwhelmed, which allows the yeast growth to take over to the point where topical over-the-counter creams are no longer effective. Essential oils with antiseptic, antibacterial, and camphoric properties like eucalyptus, oregano, and tea tree can be very effective when used in conjunction with diets low on refined sugars and refined carbohydrates.

Yeast no more blend

INGREDIENTS

- 2 drops lavender oil
- 2 drops rosemary oil
- 2 drops tea tree oil
- 2 tablespoons vinegar

DIRECTIONS

This blend can be used topically by putting the mixture in a douche and applying to the affected area at least two times a day.

Patchouli blend for men

INGREDIENTS

6 ounces warm water

5 drops patchouli oil

5 drops tea tree oil

DIRECTIONS

Mix these ingredients and use to wash the affected area well at least two times a day.

Easy flow circulation blend

Poor blood circulation can not only affect the health of your organs but also the vitality of your skin. It can lead to slow healing for small cuts and wounds and increase skin elasticity.

INGREDIENTS

10 drops geranium oil

5 drops black pepper oil

5 drops ginger oil

1.5 ounces jojoba oil

DIRECTIONS

Mix well and use by rubbing on the problem areas twice a week.

Cold and flu blend

Aromatherapy can help prevent these seasonal illnesses affecting the respiratory system.

INGREDIENTS

2 cups boiling water in a stainless steel bowl

12 drops eucalyptus oil

8 drops peppermint oil

8 drops rosemary oil

DIRECTIONS

1. Add all the ingredients into the bowl and stir.

2. Lean over the bowl with a towel over your head and inhale the steamy water until the water cools down.

3. You can also use this recipe, minus the water, in a diffuser to prevent colds and flu or blend the oils into 2 tablespoon of jojoba oil and rub on the chest and neck.

Cold sore blend

The U.S. Centers for Disease Control and Prevention (CDC) estimates that about 45 million Americans carry the herpes simplex virus. The virus, which causes cold sores, is named HSV. This results in painful and unsightly infections each year that are transmitted through person-to-person contact. The virus usually remains dormant in the body and can be awakened during stressful times or when the body's immune system is under attack and is succumbing to other infections. Using essential oils like bergamot, eucalyptus, geranium, rose, and tea tree that can boost the immune system and have antiviral and antibiotic properties can be very effective in preventing and treating flare-ups in about half the time that over-the-counter medications take.

INGREDIENTS

2 drops tea tree oil

2 drops geranium oil

4 ounces distilled water

DIRECTIONS

Use directly on the affected area three to four times a day beginning at the very first sign of a break out.

Cuts and scrapes blend

If you are the parent of young children, you know how common it is to encounter cuts and scrapes, the accompanying tears, and the subsequent days of waiting for the "boo boo" to heal. To make the waiting period less lengthy, you can use essential oils that have antiseptic or resinous properties. These include benzoic, eucalyptus, lavender, myrrh, and tea tree.

INGREDIENTS

  12 drops tea tree oil

  6 drops eucalyptus oil

  6 drops of lemon oil

  2 ounces distilled water

DIRECTIONS

Blend the oils in a spray bottle and apply on the affected area twice to three times a day.

Eczema blend

This skin condition affects children and adults, resulting in severe blistering, cracking, dryness, flaking, and itching of the skin. This condition is said to be triggered by immune system abnormalities and outside conditions such as weather, sweating, bacteria, and cosmetic products. Essential oils such as bergamot, chamomile, clary sage, lavender, litsea cubeba, and thyme can help in the development of a good immune system and treatment of the inflamed skin.

INGREDIENTS

  20 drops lavender oil

  15 drops of geranium oil

  ¾ ounce rosehip oil

  ¼ ounce litsea cubeba oil

DIRECTIONS

1. If the remedy is to be used for children younger than 5, use just 1 drop of each essential oil per year of age. Use 2 drops for children older than 5.

2. Gently massage the blend on affected areas for maximum benefit although the blend can also be used in bath water.

Exhaustion blend

When you need a little boost because of mental or physical fatigue, use oils with stimulating properties like bergamot, black pepper, cardamom, cypress, eucalyptus, frankincense, ginger, lemon, and litsea cubeba.

INGREDIENTS

15 drops frankincense oil

10 drops lemon oil

5 drops cardamom oil

DIRECTIONS

Use as a massage blend on the back, neck, and shoulders, or you can add this mixture to your bath water.

Headaches and migraine blend

As one of the most common physical ailments, headaches can be relieved by massaging 2 drops of lavender oil into the temples and at the base of the skull right where it meets the spinal cord. For migraines, blend 6 drops of peppermint oil with a tablespoon of jojoba oil and massage into temples.

Hot flashes and menopause blend

Sweeping heat, dripping perspiration, heart palpitations, night sweats, emotional upheaval, and headaches are just a few of the symptoms of this menopausal problem. These symptoms can last from a few seconds up to 15 minutes. Using essential oils to treat these symptoms provides an alternative to hormone treatments, which research has shown to put woman at increased risk for stroke, among other conditions.

INGREDIENTS

1 ounce aloe vera gel

6 drops clary sage oil

6 drops lemon oil

5 drops peppermint oil

DIRECTIONS

Using a cotton ball, dab the mixture on the face, neck, and wrists when a hot flash is coming on.

Indigestion and nausea blend

Indigestion comes when there is abnormality in the digestive track brought on by anxiety, spicy food, and other conditions. It causes stomach ache, bloating, belching, nausea and vomiting, and an acidic taste in the mouth.

INGREDIENTS

6 drops bergamot oil

6 drops chamomile oil

5 drops peppermint oil

2 Tbsp. jojoba oil

DIRECTIONS

Apply the blend on the stomach and wrists an hour before meals.

Inflammation blend

Inflammation comes as a result of tissue injury and is considered a healing process when the body fights against infection. It is characterized by pain, swelling, and redness while some conditions such as arthritis cause inflammation of the joints.

INGREDIENTS

½ ounce grapeseed oil

10 drops oregano oil

6 drops frankincense oil

6 drops lemon oil

6 drops peppermint oil

DIRECTIONS

Mix and apply directly on affected areas.

Influenza

Essential oils can help prevent and treat influenza (flu), a seasonal infection caused by a virus that infects the respiratory tract. Its symptoms include cough, fever, headache, and malaise. Use the cold and flu blend to treat these symptoms and to safeguard your home, use 1 drop each of cinnamon, cloves, eucalyptus, and pine oils in a diffuser during the flu season.

Insect repellent

Summer months offer opportunities not just to enjoy good outside weather, but they also give pesky insects an opportunity to devour your precious blood and drive you crazy. Instead of using potentially human-harmful pesticides, use specific essential oils for specific insects.

INGREDIENTS

10 drops lemongrass oil

6 drops eucalyptus oil

6 drops tea tree oil

DIRECTIONS

Using a small spray bottle, dilute the oil mixture in 8 ounces of jojoba oil, shake well, and spray directly on exposed skin.

Menstrual cramp blend

These are like mini labor pains and can sometimes last for days, with symptoms sometimes preceding and succeeding actual menstruation. They can leave a woman feeling ill, emotionally and physically, with symptoms that include backaches, headaches, and moodiness. Popping over-the-counter pills can generally help with the physical symptoms, but would it not be better to take care of the emotional and physical ailments using oils like orange and lavender?

INGREDIENTS

15 drops peppermint oil

10 drops orange oil

5 drops lavender oil

1 ounce sweet almond

DIRECTIONS

1. Mix the blend well in a small bottle and gently massage a small amount on your abdominal area, head, and back.

Sore throat

A quick gurgle of a warm water solution with a few drops of tea tree, ginger, sandalwood, or geranium essentials can help soothe sore throats. The ratio should be ½ ounce of water to three drops essential oil.

Emotional and Mental Healing

Through the sense of smell, aromatherapy can alter the way your mind and emotions work when you use them by stimulating hormonal substances in the brain. For instance, oils with sedative effects can offer relaxation by stimulating the secretion of seratonin, while oils with invigorating properties help increase energy levels because they stimulate the secretion of noradrenaline. The following represents a comprehensive list of oils you can use for various emotions.

Calming: Benzoin, chamomile, geranium, lavender, neroli, and sandalwood

Depression: Anise, basil, bergamot, chamomile, jasmine, neroli, patchouli, and ylang-ylang

Energizing: Helichrysum and rosemary

Fear: Basil, chamomile, clary sage, jasmine, marjoram, and ylang-ylang

Happiness: Cinnamon, clove, geranium, sandalwood, and ylang-ylang

Grief: Hyssop, marjoram, and rose

Indecision: Lemon, linden blossom, and patchouli

Jealousy: Rose and ylang-ylang

Loneliness: Bergamot, clary sage, frankincense, and Roman chamomile

Memory: Basil, coriander, and rosemary

Panic: Frankincense and lemongrass

Self confidence: Ginger, sandalwood, and ylang-ylang

Shock: Camphor, and neroli

Stress: Coriander, helichrysum, lemon, lemongrass, and linden blossom

Tension: Ylang-ylang

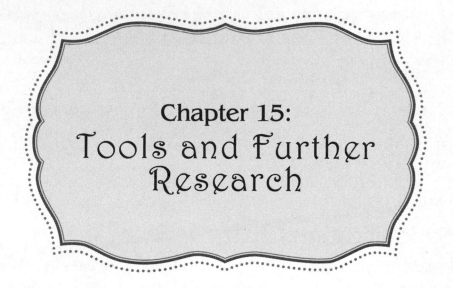

Chapter 15:
Tools and Further Research

This chapter will guide you in your quest to become a comfortable aromatherapy practitioner. Understanding the saponification (SAP) values of the oils and fats covered in this book will allow you to properly calculate the amount of lye required in each recipe. They will also allow you to spread you wings and develop your own soap recipes and essential oil blends.

In this section, you will find essential oil dilution charts and saponification charts to guide you in soap making. These are industry standard charts that can come in very handy.

Essential Oils Dilution Chart

The safest dilution for healthy adults is 2 percent, which is 2 drops of therapeutic grade essential oil for each 100 drops of carrier oil. For children, the elderly, and pregnant women use a 1 percent dilution — 1 drop of essential oils per 100 drops of carrier oil.

	Essential oil	**Carrier oil**
1 percent dilution	6 drops	1 ounce or 2 tablespoons
2 percent dilution	12 drops	2 ounces or 4 tablespoons
4 percent dilution	24 drops	4 ounces or 8 tablespoons

Saponification Charts

Calculating ingredients accurately in soap making is the most important aspect of the art. Depending on whether you are using sodium hydroxide (NaOH) for bar soap or potassium hydroxide (KOH) for liquid soap, saponification (SAP) values can help you maintain accuracy by taking the guesswork out of calculating ingredient amounts. These charts are now readily available on professional soap makers' websites for enter-as-you-go calculations, but you can also use the following formula: Ounces of carrier oil multiplied by SAP value equals amount of lye required.

Oil	Sodium Hydroxide (NaOH)	Potassium Hydroxide (KOH)
Almond	0.1367	0.1925
Apricot kernel	0.1350	0.1890
Argan	0.1340	0.1880
Avocado	0.1330	0.1862
Babassu	0.1750	0.2450
Black cumin	0.1370	0.1930
Borage	0.1339	0.1886

Oil	Sodium Hydroxide (NaOH)	Potassium Hydroxide (KOH)
Brazil nut	0.1750	0.2450
Calendula	0.1340	0.1880
Canola	0.1240	0.1736
Castor	0.1286	0.1800
Cocoa butter	0.1370	0.1918
Coconut	0.1900	0.2660
Cottonseed	0.1387	0.1954
Emu	0.1350	0.1810
Evening primrose	0.1300	0.1840
Flaxseed	0.1357	0.1900
Grapeseed	0.1265	0.1771
Hazelnut	0.1356	0.1898
Hemp	0.1345	0.1883
Jojoba	0.0690	0.0966
Kukui nut	0.1350	0.1890
Lanolin	0.0741	0.1037
Lard	0.1380	0.1932
Mango butter	0.1340	0.1890
Neem	0.1370	0.1941

Oil	Sodium Hydroxide (NaOH)	Potassium Hydroxide (KOH)
Olive	0.1340	0.1876
Ostrich	0.1335	0.1951
Palm	0.1410	0.1974
Palm kernel	0.1560	0.2184
Peanut	0.1360	0.1904
Pistachio	0.1320	0.1860
Pumpkin seed	0.1331	0.1863
Rosehip	0.1330	0.1870
Safflower	0.1360	0.1904
Sesame	0.1330	0.1862
Shea butter	0.1280	0.1792
Soybean	0.1350	0.1890
Sunflower	0.1340	0.1876
Sweet almond	0.1370	0.1930
Tallow (beef)	0.1405	0.1967
Walnut	0.1353	0.1894
Wheat germ	0.1310	0.1834

Furthering Education

Studying aromatherapy can change your life. And the best part is that you can do it in many ways. These include reading books and visiting websites on aromatherapy; taking aromatherapy classes; attending seminars; networking with experts and novices through online blogs, forums and social networking sites; and taking on volunteer, apprentice, or internship work with aromatherapy professionals.

Courses on aromatherapy

Although there is no official state government certification of aromatherapy in the United States, gaining aromatherapy knowledge and standards of practice is useful nonetheless. The National Organization for Holistic Aromatherapy, an educational, nonprofit organization dedicated to enhancing public awareness of aromatherapy benefits (**www.naha.org**) has an approved set of standards for use in aromatherapy training and features a list of approved schools offering aromatherapy courses that meet or exceed these standards. Knowledge obtained from these courses can be used in conjunction with certification from other fields that do have professional state licensure standards, such as nursing, massage therapy, and physical therapy.

Additionally, you can find courses offered locally by massage and natural care centers or enroll in online correspondence and long distance courses. Make sure you do your homework before spending any money on these courses, especially because courses and materials can cost several hundreds to thousands of dollars. Visit websites, make contact over the telephone and ask questions, and even search the Better Business Bureau website (**www.bbb.org**) for any consumer complaints. Try to select courses offered by entities that follow NAHA standards even when they are not on the NAHA approved list of schools.

Suppliers

Finding a good supplier of all-natural, therapeutic-grade essential oils is important to ensure you are receiving the oils that will offer you the most healing potential. By doing your homework, knowing your products, talking to more experienced aromatherapy professionals or practitioners, and dealing locally, you can avoid pitfalls. When it is not feasible to deal locally, visit the websites of registered organizations such as The Alliance of International Aromatherapists (**www.alliance-aromatherapists.org**) and find suggested supplier lists.

For soap making supplies, Bramble Berry, located in Washington state and online at **www.brambleberry.com**, is a good place to start. The company has a wide selection of natural and organic ingredients and equipment.

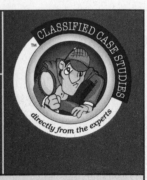

CASE STUDY: SHAKOOR'S MERCHANDISE

Dawud and Mahasin Shakoor
319 North 2nd Street
Richmond, Va. 23219
804-644-4494
dmshakoor@aol.com

Mahasin Shakoor, vice president of Shakoor's Merchandise, a retailer of many natural goods, including essential oils, carrier oils, soaps, and other health products, suggests that once you find a good supplier, make sure that they are also consistent.

"You do not want to use any supplier that will decide soon afterwards, to change the products they supply," she said. "You want them to be consistent and supply the same products for years to come."

Mahasin Shakoor and her husband, Dawud, have been selling a consistent array of health products for more than a decade. She said they got started after realizing that chemical-based products and pharmaceuticals may claim to be healing, but sometimes have side effects that are worse than whatever illness you sought the treatment for in the first place.

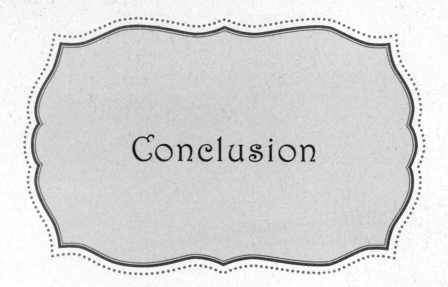

Conclusion

The information in this book is good reference material, but it does not include everything there is to know about aromatherapy. Furthering your education by reading other specialized literature and maybe taking aromatherapy courses can turn you into a walking aromatherapy and essential oils specialist and open the doors to a healthy, all-natural life that is good for your mind and body.

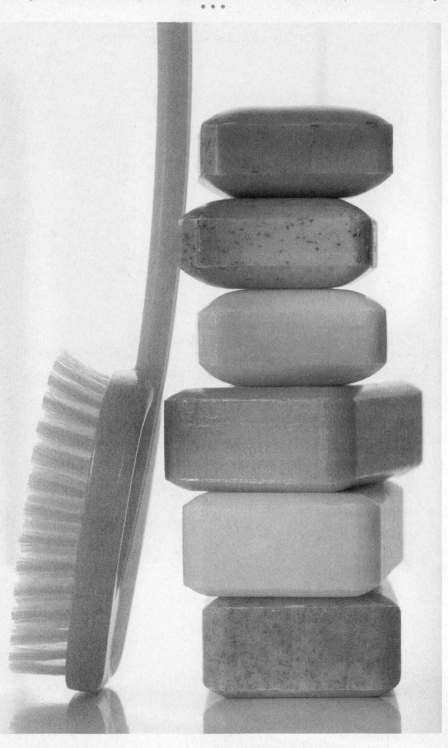

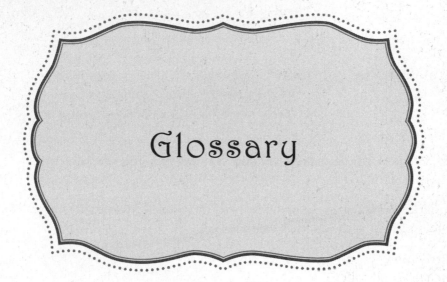

Glossary

Absolute: an oil that results from introducing chemical solvents to plant matter, such as leaves or flowers, during the extraction process

Alkali: lye made from wood ash

Aromatic synergy: blending two or more essential oils together

Base note: a scent characterized by a scent that lasts for several hours or even days

Base: cold-pressed, plant-based oils from vegetables, nuts, or seeds

Carbon dioxide extraction: using extraction equipment to pressurize and turn carbon dioxide into a liquid that is then used to steam distill essential oils

Enfleurage: saturating flowers with vegetable oils to release their essences

Expression: using high pressure to squeeze out plant essences

Flash point: the lowest temperature at which liquid can vaporize into air, forming a mixture capable of igniting

Hydrodistillation: extracting essential oils by tightly packing and fully submerging plant matter in a still's kettle and heating the plant to 212 degrees to produce a soup-like product

Lipids: compounds such as oils and waxes that do not dissolve in water

Lye: a caustic substance that causes chemical reactions necessary to make soap

Lye discounting: a soap maker can either add extra oil to a soap recipe while keeping the amount of lye the same, or reduce the amount of lye in the soap while keeping the oil the same; this helps produce soaps that are moisturizing

Middle note: oils that have a scent that lasts two to four hours before evaporating

Poultices: moist preparations made out of an herb's flowers that are macerated in alcohol for at least one week

Processing: separating the carrier oils from their hosts

Reaching trace: the point in soap making when a mixture reaches a pudding-like consistency

Reverse osmosis: a process where hard water passes through a membrane that removes chemicals

Saponification: splitting oils or fats into their natural parts (fatty acids and glycerin)

Sequestering: allowing a mixture to sit undisturbed

Solvent extraction: using chemicals such as alcohol to saturate dainty flowers, allowing them to release their essential oils

Steam distillation: the process of placing fresh or dried plant matter into a device similar to a pressure cooker to extract essential oils

Still: a device similar to a pressure cooker that is used in steam distillation

Super fatting: adding extra oil at trace so the resulting soap is very nourishing

Tocopherals: stable lipids that are known to resist oxidization, which can cause oils to go rancid

Top note: oils that evaporate quickly

Volatile: a quality that makes oils evaporate quickly

Bibliography

"A Wise Man's Remedy for Bladder Cancer" Medical News Today, March 18, 2009.

Acne Cures Reviewed. **www.approvedcures.com**. Accessed September 29, 2010.

Anatolian Treasures. **www.av-at.com**. Accessed September 29, 2010.

Aqua de Luna: Unique Fragrances of the World. **www.aquadeluna.com**. Accessed September 29, 2010.

Aromatics International. **www.aromaticsinternational.com**. Accessed September 29, 2010.

Beauty Without Cruelty. **www.beautywithoutcruelty.com**. Accessed September 29, 2010.

Blumenfield, Larry. *The Big Book of Relaxation: Simple Techniques to Control the Excess Stress in Your Life.* Roslyn, NY: The Relaxation Company. 1994.

Botanical.com. **www.botanical.com**. Accessed September 29, 2010.

Cavitch, Susan Miller. *The Natural Soap Book: Making Herbal and Vegetable-Based Soaps*. North Adams, MA: Storey Publishing. 1995.

Cavitch, Susan Miller. *The Soapmaker's Companion: A Comprehensive Guide with Recipes, Techniques & Know-How*. North Adams, MA: Storey Publishing. 1997.

Coss, Melinda. *The Handmade Soap Book*. North Adams, MA: Storey Publishing. 1998.

Dodt, Colleen K. *The Essential Oils Book: Creating personal Blends for Mind and Body*. North Adams, MA: Storey Publishing. 1996.

Eden Botanicals. **www.edenbotanicals.com**. Accessed September 29, 2010.

Essencial Dreams. **www.essentialdreams.com**. Accessed September 29, 2010.

Keville, Kathi and Mindy Green. *Aromatherapy: A Complete Guide to the Healing Art*. Freedom, California: Crossing Press. 1995.

Korkina, L.G. "Phenylpropanoids as Naturally Occurring Antioxidants: From Plant Defense to Human Health" *Cellular and Molecular Biology*. 2007.

Melaleuca Business Builder. **www.rmbarry.com.** Accessed September 29, 2010.

Miller's Homemade Soap Page. **www.millersoap.com.** Accessed September 29, 2010.

National Association for Holistic Aromatherapy. **www.naha.org.** Accessed September 29, 2010.

Purdue University Horticulture and Landscape Agriculture. **www.hort.purdue. edu**. Accessed September 29, 2010.

Romer, Tammie and Tiffany Richards-Thibodeaux. "Aromatherapy Eases Addiction Recovery." Alternative Health, Jan./Feb. 2007.

Wellness.com. **www.wellness.com**. Accessed September 29, 2010.

Author Biography

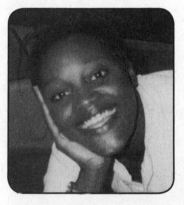

This is Marlene Jones' first full-length book but she has been writing professionally since 2001 right after leaving journalism school. Over the years, she has written pieces on a variety of subjects, focusing especially on issues of health and wellness related to low-income and minority communities.

Her interest in all things natural sparked in 2005 after the birth of her first child and after being prompted by her older sister's quests to eliminate synthetic and chemical-laden products from her diet and cosmetics. Marlene's upbringing in Kenya is also a major source for learning how to be one with nature. She continues to learn the many different aspects of natural living and uses her platform as a journalist to inform others about the benefits available.

When Marlene is not writing and researching, she is parenting her precious three babies, dabbling in politics, traveling the world, and working hard to be active.

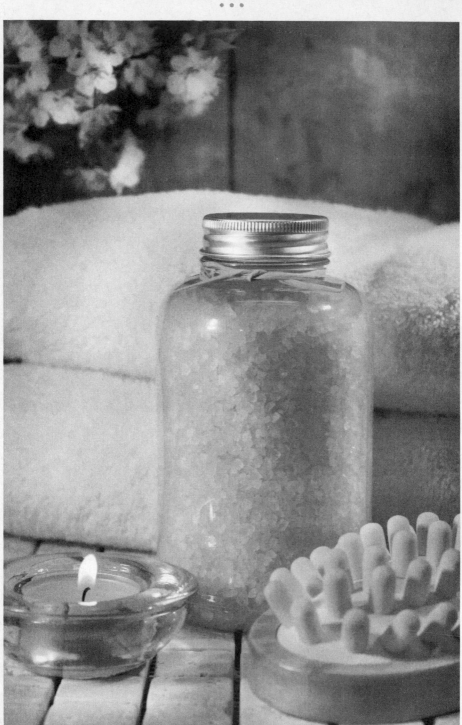

Index